Living with
head injury

Living with

Each book in this series deals with a medical or psychological condition. It contains background and medical information on causes and symptoms and explains treatment in some detail – both practical (drug treatments, surgery) and psychological (self-help, home care, social implications)

Series editors: John Riordan and Bob Whitmore

Living with stress and anxiety
Bob Whitmore

Living with breast cancer and mastectomy
Nicholas Tarrier

Living with dementia
John Riordan and Bob Whitmore

Living with back pain
Helen Parker and Chris J. Main

Living with stroke
Paul King

Living with anorexia and bulimia
James Moorey

Living with tinnitus
David W. Rees and Simon D. Smith

Living with grief and mourning
James Moorey

Living with head injury
M. D. van den Broek, W. Shady and M. J. Coyne

Living with
head injury

M. D. van den Broek,
W. Schady & M. J. Coyne

Manchester University Press

Manchester and New York

Distributed exclusively in the USA and Canada
by St Martin's Press

Published by Manchester University Press
Oxford Road, Manchester M13 9NR, UK
and Room 400, 175 Fifth Avenue, New York, NY 10010, USA

Distributed exclusively in the USA and Canada
by St Martin's Press, Inc.,
175 Fifth Avenue, New York, NY 10010, USA

British Library Cataloguing-in-Publication Data
A catalogue record for this book is available from the British Library

Library of Congress Cataloging-in-Publication Data
Broek, M. D. van den, 1959-
    Living with head injury / M. D. van den Broek, W. Schady, and M. J. Coyne.
        p.   cm. — (Living with)
    Includes bibliographical references.
    ISBN 0-7190-4189-9. — ISBN 0-7190-4190-2 (pbk.)
    1. Brain damage. I. Schady, Wolfgang J. L. II. Coyne, M. J. III. Title
IV. Series.
    RC387.5.B76   1995
    362.1'97481—dc20   95-3490
                                                   CIP

ISBN 0 7190 4189 9 *hardback*
ISBN 0 7190 4190 2 *paperback*

First published 1995

99 98 97 96 95   10 9 8 7 6 5 4 3 2 1

Typeset in New Century Schoolbook
by Koinonia, Manchester
Printed in Great Britain
by Bell & Bain Ltd, Glasgow

Contents

1 Head injury: the silent epidemic

Head injury is the most common cause of brain damage in young adults. Approximately 4,000 people die each year in England and Wales as a result of a head injury, and the Royal College of Physicians has estimated that in Britain approximately 7,500 people suffer a severe head injury every year. As a result, one family in three hundred has a disabled survivor of head trauma. The picture in America is very similar. There, head trauma is the most common cause of death after cancer and heart disease, and it has been estimated that over two million people annually suffer traumatic brain injuries. If the number of head injuries is compared with other conditions, they are found to be much more common than strokes or tumours and forty times more common than spinal cord injuries. Clearly brain trauma is a major health problem in Western countries, although its importance has only been recognised relatively recently by health service planners and governments: small wonder that it has been called the 'silent epidemic'.

Although most head injuries are mild and do not cause any lasting disability, significant numbers of people are left with persistent problems. Survivors may have physical injuries such as difficulty moving their limbs, loss of taste and smell or blurred or double vision. There may be long-term complications such as fits (epilepsy), severe headaches or dizziness. As well as these medical complaints there may be psychological changes affecting the person's character and mood, such as irritability and rages. Alternatively they may have difficulty motivating themselves, feel depressed and lack drive. They may say or do embarrassing or inappropriate things in public, such as talking about personal or sexual matters. There may also be changes in what are termed a person's cognitive abilities, such as their capacity to think clearly, reason or remember. People who have sustained a severe head injury commonly suffer from both medical and psychological disabilities. However, even after injuries from which a person makes a good or excellent physical recovery – and this occurs in about ninety per cent of cases – there may nevertheless be significant psychological problems. These physical and psychological problems can have a considerable impact on a person's ability to live independently, get back to work and lead a normal life. The sufferer may have to cope with physical limitations and psychological changes, as well as other problems such as financial difficulties and changes in relationships, and adjust to a different future.

Head injury affects not only the person who has been injured but many other people as well. Wives, husbands, partners, children and parents may all find their lives changed. The injury is invariably a sudden and unexpected event, perhaps the result of a car crash or fall, and the victim may have been leading a healthy and normal life one day, and be irrevocably changed the next. The family has to adjust to this sudden and traumatic event and later may have to look after someone with a significant disability. The strain of caring for a head-injured person can often be considerable and affect the family's own physical and mental health.

Causes of head injury

By far the most common cause of head injury is road traffic accidents when people suffer a blow to their head in the course of a car crash or motorbike accident. In a car crash the driver or passengers may be thrown violently against the windscreen, dashboard or each other, and so suffer blows to the head and face as well as to other parts of the body. The legal requirement to wear seatbelts has significantly reduced the mortality rate from car crashes and also resulted in a reduction in the incidence of brain injury; nevertheless car accidents remain one of the most common causes. In motorbike accidents the driver may be catapulted onto the road or some other obstacle and at that point incur head injuries. Accidents in the home such as falling down the stairs and industrial accidents at work are the next most common cause. In America, where guns are readily available, gunshot wounds to the face and head are an additional factor, although, as might be expected, such injuries are far less common in Britain where there are comparatively fewer guns. Nevertheless violence does play a role, and fights or attempted strangulation can result in brain damage. While it is true to say that anyone can sustain a head injury, they are much more likely to happen to some people than to others. For instance, men are much more likely to suffer a head injury than women: for every woman with brain trauma there are two or three men. Young people are much more at risk: approximately seventy per cent of head injuries occur in people under the age of thirty, and the majority are under the age of twenty. It is also known that people who are unemployed or from lower socio-economic classes are more likely to receive a head injury. Alcohol has an important role to play: when admitted to hospital a significant proportion of victims are found to have been drinking and have exceeded the legal limit. There are even certain days of the week and times of day when head injuries are more likely to occur, these being Friday and Saturday evenings before midnight. We can draw these details together to obtain a picture of the typical head-injured person; he is a teenager or young adult who has been out for an evening with his friends, in the course of which he has driven or been a passenger in a car or on a motorbike which has then been involved in a collision.

What happens during head injury?

How do blows to the head cause the brain to be damaged? What happens is that in, say, a car crash the victim is suddenly and violently thrown forward or upwards and invariably strikes parts of the car, such as the roof or dashboard. Depending on the speed and angle at which the car was struck, the head, and consequently the brain inside, will be subjected to strong rotational forces which cause the brain's nerve fibres to stretch and shear. If the person hits something the head will come to an abrupt stop, but the brain inside will not and it moves forwards and backwards inside the skull causing lacerations and contusions. Doctors distinguish between open and closed head injuries. The term **open head injury** is used when a person has suffered a blow to the head as a result of which the skull is penetrated and the brain underneath is exposed. A gunshot wound would, for instance, belong to this category. **Closed head injury**, on the other hand, refers to when the head has received a blow, but the skull remains intact. Unfortunately, even though there may be no damage to the cranium, this does not necessarily mean that the person has not suffered brain damage, and one should not think that he or she has suffered a less serious injury.

The term 'head injury' perhaps implies that sufferers are a relatively uniform group of people with similar problems. In reality, however, although they share the fact that they have had a blow to the head, they can differ enormously in terms of the problems they subsequently experience. Some people are left with nothing in the way of physical disability, although they may have mild psychological problems such as a tendency to be irritable or a slight loss of drive. Others have major physical handicaps and need continual nursing care, as well as serious behavioural problems such as violent and aggressive outbursts. How then can we distinguish between these different kinds of injuries? The Medical Disability Society classified head injuries on the basis of the duration of any loss of consciousness and the length of what is known as the **post-traumatic amnesia**. It may be helpful to define what is meant by this term. After a head injury a person may be confused and unable to take in information properly and his or her working memory may be affected: this is post-traumatic amnesia and it is the time between the original injury and the restitution of a person's continuous memory. The Medical Disability Society has drawn up the following system of classification:

- **Minor brain injury:** an injury causing unconsciousness for 15 minutes or less.
- **Moderate brain injury**: a head injury resulting in a loss of consciousness for more than 15 minutes and less than 6 hours, and a period of post-traumatic amnesia of less than 24 hours.
- **Severe brain injury**: loss of consciousness for 6 or more hours or post-traumatic amnesia of 24 hours or more.
- **Very severe brain injury**: when the injury causes loss of consciousness for 48 hours or more or post-traumatic amnesia of a week or more.

In other words, the longer the loss of consciousness or post-traumatic amnesia, the more serious the injury and the greater the degree of damage to the brain. The majority of people have relatively minor injuries – for example, as a result of playing sports when they briefly knock themselves out. This may not result in any lasting neurological problems such as muscle weakness or dizziness, although it may bring about short-lived psychological changes such as feelings of depression or impaired concentration. As might be expected, long-term physical problems such as fits, muscle weakness and visual disorders, as well as incapacitating psychological changes such as profound forgetfulness, are increasingly likely to be associated with more severe injuries. However, while this is true as a rule, one of the perplexing things about head injury is that there are many exceptions, and some people who have serious injuries escape relatively unaffected, whereas others who have received apparently less serious injuries do not.

Effects of head injury

- **Physical**: e.g., Headaches, muscle weakness or paralysis, double vision, incontinence
- **Emotional**: e.g., depression, anxiety, grief
- **Behavioural**: e.g., inappropriate behaviour, rages
- **Cognitive**: e.g., forgetfulness, poor concentration, impaired reasoning
- **Family**: e.g., stress of caring, changed relationships

Hospital staff: who they are and what they do

Only a small proportion of head-injured people – approximately twenty per cent – are actually admitted to hospital and most either do not go to hospital or are treated by their GP. Many are examined at an Accident and Emergency Department where cuts and broken bones are treated and they are then discharged without being admitted to a hospital ward. Of those who are admitted, an even smaller number are seen in specialist neurosurgical units and most are treated on general medical wards. Depending on the precise nature of the problems they experience, head-injured people may need to see what can be a bewildering number of different staff. In the following chapters we will look in detail at how care is organised, medical tests and examinations, complications which may arise, and what treatments may be necessary and why. Here we will look at the members of the hospital team and explain who they are and what they do.

Medical staff

When someone is admitted to hospital he or she is placed under the care of a consultant and a team of junior medical staff. Most treatment and investigations are in fact provided by the junior staff or other professionals such as nurses, although this is always under the direction of the consultant. While a person may remain under the overall care of one consultant, such as a neurosurgeon, he or she may see many different consultants and junior doctors from different specialties. Each of these doctors is specialised in a particular field, such as the treatment of disorders of the nervous system (neurologist) or injuries to the bones or joints (orthopaedic surgeon). They may be asked to advise on a specific problem and recommend a course of treatment. As progress is made, responsibility for overseeing care may be transferred from one consultant to another: when admitted as an emergency, for instance, a person may be managed by a surgeon, but later a specialist in rehabilitation medicine may take charge.

Nursing staff

Nurses play a vital role in treating head injury. They are the only professionals who are with the patient day and night and consequently they know best how he or she is progressing and can provide invaluable emotional support to patient and family. The nurses observe the patient, and ensure that he or she is getting adequate nutrition and is properly positioned so that breathing is not hampered. The patient will be moved regularly to ensure that complications such as bedsores do not occur. The nurses conduct regular assessments, implement treatments and rehabilitation, and liaise closely with the medical staff.

Clinical psychologist

The clinical psychologist, or neuropsychologist as he or she is sometimes called, is concerned with assessing and treating the psychological effects of head injury. The clinical psychologist may administer tests of memory, concentration or logical reasoning to ascertain if these abilities have been affected, and then recommend strategies to overcome or circumvent problems, as well as advise on future rehabilitation goals. He or she will also assess any emotional or behavioural problems and recommend appropriate treatments.

Occupational therapist

The occupational therapist assesses how well a person is able to look after himself or herself, and cope with essential matters such as washing, dressing, cooking and managing money. In other words, the occupational therapist helps retrain the person's skills so as to maximise his or her level of independence. This may be done by setting goals in rehabilitation, and then organising a daily programme of activities which stimulate the person's concentration and help restore his or her planning skills and capacity to initiate and organise activities. The occupational therapist may visit the patient's home before he or she leaves hospital and recommend aids and adaptations that need to be made.

Speech therapist

Brain damage can affect a person's ability to produce and understand speech, and there may be difficulties with swallowing and articulation. The speech therapist is specialised in assessing communication problems, and will conduct a detailed examination to determine their exact nature and severity. This information is then conveyed to other members of the team as well as to the family, to help them better understand the person's problems. The therapist may recommend ways of circumventing difficulties, exercises to improve articulation, or communication aids.

Physiotherapist

Problems with movement and mobility are not uncommon following severe head injuries. Physiotherapists are specialised in assessing patients' capacity for movement and balance and advising on how to handle and position limbs, sit and stand. They will recommend and initiate exercises to increase mobility, reduce pain and improve independent movement, as well as advise on procedures to prevent complications such as painful limbs and deformities. They may recommend the use of various aids such as wheelchairs.

Social worker

A social worker is often the key person who acts as a bridge between the hospital and the home and hence communicates between the staff and the family. He or she will discuss with the family the post-discharge arrangements and advise on issues such as benefit entitlements and financial matters, respite care, work and retraining, and a range of other practical matters. The social worker can monitor how the family is coping and provide essential support while recovery is taking place.

The doctors, nurses and other professionals meet regularly, usually weekly, at ward rounds to discuss how each patient is progressing and make plans for the future. Most teams will want to be in regular contact with the family to keep them informed of progress, and in time discuss arrangements for discharge. Family members may be asked to go along to ward rounds to discuss with the team their hopes and plans for the future. Members of the team will also liaise with other bodies as needed, such as the patient's employers, school or college. When the patient is medically stable this is often the time when plans are made for them to move on and leave hospital. Usually this is not an all-or-nothing event and often the head-injured person starts by going home for just a weekend to see how things go and to regain confidence away from the security of the hospital environment. The family may also need time to adjust to the new situation, and this is often best achieved by a step-by-step approach. The eventual discharge from hospital care does not necessarily mean that there will be no more problems, and indeed for many people and their families this is the beginning of a long period of learning and adjustment. Nor is it necessarily an indication that no further progress can be made, and that any psychological or physical problems are unchangeable. As we will see in subsequent chapters, there are many practical steps that can be taken to reduce or minimise these problems and so make living with head injury easier.

Who this book is for

As we have seen, head trauma may affect not just the person who sustains the injury, but also other people such as family, friends and carers. In the following chapters we will describe the main effects of head injury and some practical steps to overcome or minimise them. This is intended to be of help not only to those who have had a head injury, but also to relatives and carers. Sometimes the effects of head injury are such that the injured person either cannot or is unwilling to accept that they have any problems: in such circumstances it may be the carers who will find this book most useful and we have therefore included a chapter on the problems they experience. We have tried to address the main areas that are often of interest to injured people and their families – medical, psychological and legal issues. Inevitably, however, there will be gaps, as the effects of head trauma are varied and the needs of injured people and their families are invariably complex. At the end of the book is a list of the addresses of organisations and agencies which can be of help in providing more information and support.

2 Hospital care after head injury

Head injuries vary enormously in their severity. The majority are minor and do not give rise to concern. Unless complications set in they do not cause any damage to the brain. Those that are more serious have a number of effects for which various terms are used. It may be of value to list and define these terms, since they are frequently used by doctors and appear in records, medico-legal reports, chapters in this book and other books.

- A **laceration** is a tear in the scalp, the coverings of the brain (the meninges) or the brain itself.
- **Cerebral contusion** means bruising of the brain. Such contusions may be on the surface or deep inside the brain and there is often a little blood within them.
- An **intracranial haematoma** is a blood clot inside the head.
- **Cerebral concussion** is a transient disorder of the functions of the brain, caused by a blow to the head and resulting in loss of consciousness, confusion or forgetfulness.

Whether or not a blow to the head has any of these effects depends not only on the force of the blow but on the point of impact, the position of the head, the age of the injured person and other factors which we do not fully understand. An apparently insignificant bang on the head in an elderly person may result in serious bleeding in the brain, whereas a child may fall from a considerable height onto his or her head and walk away, none the worse for it. By and large, however, the level of consciousness in the aftermath of the accident and the duration of post-traumatic amnesia provide a measure of the severity of the head injury, as has been mentioned in the previous chapter.

A number of scales are used to assess the level of consciousness in a patient admitted to a hospital casualty department after head trauma. A person may be fully alert and orientated; he or she may be drowsy and lethargic; stuporose, that is to say, he or she lapses into sleep when not disturbed; or in a state of coma. The depth of coma can be judged from a person's response to spoken commands and to a painful stimulus, such as squeezing a finger. One of the most widely used grading systems is the Glasgow Coma Scale (GCS), which assigns a score depending on the injured person's level of responsiveness.

Eye opening	4 – spontaneous
	3 – to speech
	2 – to pain
	1 – nil
Best verbal response	5 – orientated
	4 – confused
	3 – inappropriate words
	2 – incomprehensible sounds
	1 – nil
Best motor response	6 – obeys commands
	5 – localises pain
	4 – withdraws limb
	3 – abnormal flexion
	2 – extension
	1 – nil

The scores for the three components of the test are added and a value is obtained which varies from 3 (worst) to 15 (best). In the early stages after a head injury a GCS score is often obtained at hourly intervals to assess if someone is improving or deteriorating.

Concussion and loss of consciousness may result from a blow to any part of the head, provided it is forceful enough. These are what are called the **diffuse** effects of a head injury. However, a head injury may also have **focal** effects, that is, it may produce damage to localised areas. On the scalp it may cause a laceration, or the skull below may be fractured. The underlying brain may be focally injured causing contusion, or a blood vessel may be torn, resulting in a blood clot (an intracranial haematoma). Interestingly, patients in a coma after a road traffic accident are more likely to have diffuse cerebral injury and less likely to have focal damage than those with a head injury sustained during an assault. Not all focal injuries occur immediately below the point of impact. So-called 'contre-coup' contusions occur in that part of the brain opposite the site of impact due to a sudden shift in the brain's position within the skull (a sort of whiplash injury to the brain). This is, for instance, how the olfactory nerves, which are located underneath the front parts of the brain (and are responsible for our sense of smell), are sometimes damaged by blows to the back of the head.

In order to understand the effects of an injury it is helpful to know about the normal functions of each part of the brain. The brain is comprised of two halves, or **cerebral hemispheres**, each of which is made up of four parts, the frontal, parietal, temporal and occipital lobes. The right hemisphere deals with functions on the left side of the body, and vice versa so that, for example, your right arm is controlled by the left side of your brain, while your left arm is controlled by the right half. The **frontal lobes** are thought to be involved in planning, sequencing, goal selection and other supervisory or executive functions. They also have an important role in the mediation of movement. The left one also deals with speech in right-handed individuals and in about seventy-five per cent of people who are left-handed. The **parietal lobes** are important for normal sensation. The **temporal lobes** process hearing and memory, and the **occipital lobes** at the back of the brain are concerned with vision. Lastly, the **hindbrain** (or brainstem) deals with balance, sleep and control of the internal organs.

An early consideration for the doctor looking after a patient with a head injury is to establish whether there has been damage to the skull and the layers which surround the brain which are called the meninges. There are three forms of skull fracture: a **linear** fracture, which is a simple crack in the bone; a **depressed** fracture, where one or a few fragments of bone are pushed in towards the cranial cavity; and a **comminuted** fracture, in which multiple small bony fragments are formed and there is usually very obvious deformity of the skull. In the previous chapter we mentioned that doctors distinguish between 'open' and 'closed' head injuries. A head injury is said to be 'closed' when the meninges which cover the brain are intact. The meninges in fact consist of three layers, of which the outermost (the dura) is the toughest. If a skull fracture is accompanied by a tear in the dura, the head injury is classed as 'open'. In these circumstances the fluid which bathes the brain (which is called cerebrospinal fluid or CSF) may leak out and infection may make its way into the skull. All of these are important points doctors have to consider when planning the treatment of a head-injured patient.

The age of the injured person also has a bearing on the severity of the head injury. Elderly people have more fragile bones, whereas a baby's brain is better protected by the flexibility of the skull bones and the greater amount of fluid bathing the brain. Nevertheless, it has been estimated that about one child in ten suffers a blow to the head of sufficient force to cause loss of consciousness at some time or other. Boys are more likely than girls to suffer a head injury and the highest incidence is in the summer. Falls, road accidents and assault are the commonest causes of head injury in children, whereas in adults road traffic accidents by far outstrip the other two. Fortunately, children have a very adaptable brain and their long-term recovery is often better than might be expected from an assessment of their condition immediately after the injury.

Clinical features

When a person has had a head injury, the doctor will want to establish from witnesses whether the person was conscious and coherent at the scene of the accident. Coma from the moment of impact implies what is called **primary** brain damage, while subsequent deterioration in the level of consciousness suggests that a complication has developed (**secondary** brain damage). After a blow to the head, be it at work or on the roads, a person may be taken to hospital for an examination, although as mentioned in the previous chapter many people do not receive any specific treatment. Nevertheless, this is a sensible precaution, not only from the point of view of treatment but also for the purpose of documentation in case there are medico-legal implications. The ambulance staff will monitor the patient's condition and convey their observations to the medical staff at the hospital.

Having arrived in the Accident and Emergency Department, the patient will initially be assessed by a specialist nurse, who assigns a level of urgency to each patient. This is done in order to ensure that the most seriously ill (not only from the head injury point of view) are dealt with first. Their level of consciousness will be determined and, if it is impaired, a coma scale score will probably be obtained, in the way mentioned earlier. If the patient is awake he or she will be asked whether he or she is in pain and whether there are any other symptoms. Enquiries will be made about whether he or she has been drinking alcohol, since intoxication may cause confusion and sleepiness which cloud the assessment of the head injury. An examination will then take place, attention being focused initially on the vital signs such as pulse and blood pressure and later on to individual parts of the body.

Breathing

If the head-injured person is unconscious it is very important to observe his or her breathing pattern. If he or she has difficulty breathing, the mouth and throat will be checked for obstructions and a free passage of air will be ensured. He or she will have been transported in the recovery position (i.e., lying on his or her side) to prevent choking on the tongue and to avoid inhalation of vomit. An abnormal breathing rhythm may be a pointer to brain damage. Rapid shallow breathing can be expected from someone who is in pain or anxious, as well as from the presence of chest injuries. Irregular breathing in an unconscious head-injured patient often signifies raised pressure inside the head. Such a finding may prompt the doctors to pass a tube into the person's airway and connect him or her to a machine called a ventilator to assist breathing.

Vital signs

All patients will have their pulse and blood pressure checked on admission to hospital. Falling blood pressure and rising pulse would alert the staff to the possibility of internal bleeding. A large amount of blood can be lost into the abdomen because of its flexible walls. Tears in solid organs such as the liver or spleen are particularly dangerous. Bleeding into the chest is less common unless there are extensive rib fractures. As regards the head, when there is bleeding inside the skull problems do not arise from the actual blood loss but from compression of the brain, since the skull, unlike the abdomen, cannot expand. The resulting rise in pressure in the head may in fact cause the opposite effect to that expected from blood loss, namely an increase in blood pressure and a fall in the pulse rate. This is a well-known sign of deterioration in a head-injured patient which will trigger urgent investigation and treatment.

Conscious level

We have already referred to the assessment of the level of consciousness which will be carried out as soon as the injured person arrives in the Accident and Emergency Department. How often a coma scale score is obtained depends on the seriousness of the patient's condition and on the nursing resources available. In an unconscious patient it will be checked, together with the vital signs, every fifteen minutes for the first few hours; hourly once a stable pattern has been observed and every four hours while recovery is taking place. A fall in the Glasgow Coma Scale score may be a pointer to secondary brain damage due to the development of some complication.

The pupils

A great deal of attention will be paid by doctors to the pupils, since they too can reflect the pressure inside the head. When pressure increases there may be compression of one of the nerves which control the pupils, resulting in them becoming enlarged. At the same time the movements of the eye may be disrupted, but this is less easy to ascertain in an unconscious patient. The pupils are therefore checked for their size, symmetry and response to light. A larger pupil on one side, with loss of the normal response to light, is a serious development in this context. When both pupils are enlarged, the pressure inside the head has reached such levels that the situation is critical.

The scalp

If the doctor detects a scalp laceration he or she will feel gently for signs of a skull fracture. The deeper the laceration, the more likely it is that the skull has been injured. Bleeding may be quite profuse and will be stemmed by stitching and dressing the wound. There may be a bruise without a break in the skin. Its position does not necessarily indicate the point of impact. For example, bruising around the eyes and behind the ears may develop in fractures of the skull base.

The eyes

If there has been a blow to the face the eyelids may be so swollen that one or both eyes are closed. This looks very alarming but it tends to subside within two to three weeks. The movements of the eyes are controlled by several muscles, which in turn are supplied by three nerves. Bruising within the eye sockets may make it difficult for an eye to move and if the other eye can move normally double vision will ensue. By and large, such bruising resolves itself fairly soon without serious long-term consequences. On the other hand, if double vision results from damage to one of the cranial nerves recovery will take longer and may be incomplete. Some patients are given a patch to cover one eye for at least part of the day and thus avoid double vision.

The ears and nose
If the nose is broken there will be difficulty breathing through it. Equally, a tear in the eardrum will cause local pain and impaired hearing. Bleeding from the ear or nose merits further consideration. In the early stages after the head injury it may simply stem from a small laceration. If it persists it is often a pointer to a leak of blood mixed with cerebrospinal fluid (CSF), which, as we mentioned earlier, is the fluid which surrounds the brain. Loss of CSF is more evident when the discharge from the ear (which is called otorrhoea) or nose (which is called rhinorrhoea) is clear, as CSF is normally colourless. In a head-injured person this observation suggests that there has been a fracture of the base of the skull which allows the fluid to escape.

The face
The small nerves which run across the upper and lower rims of the eye socket are particularly vulnerable to injury. When they are damaged a small patch of skin on the forehead or cheek may become numb. Later this numbness turns to tingling or hypersensitivity. Weakness of one side of the face may result from an injury either to the brain itself, in which case it is usually accompanied by weakness of the arm and leg on the same side, or to the facial nerve. This nerve may be damaged early on by a skull base fracture, or as a delayed effect of a haemorrhage or local swelling. The facial weakness tends to be less pronounced (and it spares the forehead muscles) when the damage is in the brain than when the nerve itself is affected.

The neck
Neck stiffness and pain are common features of a whiplash injury which often accompanies a head injury. Severe pain at this site raises the possibility of a fracture of the cervical spine

(neck). The neck may also be stiff when there has been bleeding on the surface of the brain, which irritates the meninges.

The limbs

A head-injured person may have no complaints about his or her arms and legs but they will nevertheless be examined, not only for signs of direct trauma but also for evidence of nervous system damage. As mentioned earlier, the right half or hemisphere of the brain controls the left side of the body and vice versa. This means that weakness on one side, often with exaggerated reflexes, can lead the doctor to diagnose damage in the opposite hemisphere. When all four limbs are weak or paralysed, the site of damage is more likely to be in the upper spinal cord or the brainstem.

Complications

In the aftermath of a head injury there may be a deterioration in the patient's condition, often after an interval when he or she is quite lucid. This heralds the onset of a complication, and it is precisely because such complications have to be recognised and treated that coma scores are obtained regularly when the patient is admitted to hospital. Any patient whose level of consciousness deteriorates is usually considered to have a blood clot on the brain until proven otherwise.

Extradural haematoma

An extradural (or epidural) haematoma is a collection of blood on the surface of the brain but outside the dura (in other words, between the dura and the skull bone). There is a fracture of the skull in the great majority of sufferers, often in the temples. Bleeding takes place from blood vessels just inside the skull, and the haematoma grows as it gradually strips the dura from the skull. Usually the haemorrhage begins immediately after the head injury, but it only becomes obvious that it is present when there is significant compression of the brain.

It is not only the size of the clot that matters but its speed of development. An extradural haematoma is a particularly dangerous complication because the torn blood vessels tend to be arteries, which carry blood under much more pressure than

veins. Bleeding is therefore brisk and the brain will be compressed more rapidly than if the source of blood loss is from
veins. It is very rare for such a clot to cause symptoms in the
first hour after the head injury. However, after that the patient
becomes increasingly drowsy, irritable or restless. There may
be vomiting, slowing of the pulse, weakness down one side of the
body, abnormalities of the pupils and disturbed eye movements.
When the eyes do not move in unison the sufferer, if awake,
complains of double vision. These features all suggest that
there has been a build-up of pressure inside the head from the
expanding clot. If not acted upon urgently this can be fatal.

Subdural haematoma
This is a collection of blood underneath the dura, which is the
layer surrounding the brain. While to the lay person the distinc-
tion between extradural and subdural haematomas may seem
pointless, they behave differently and their long-term outcome
is not the same. Subdural haematomas are usually brought
about by the rupture of small veins. The rate of blood loss is
usually slower than when arteries are torn, though an acute
life-threatening subdural haematoma may occur when a larger
vessel is involved. There is less resistance to the spread of blood
below the dura and the clot can therefore cover the whole of a
hemisphere of the brain. Sometimes a subdural haematoma
occurs at a distance from the site of impact due to a shearing or
whiplash effect.

Subdural haematomas are uncommon immediately after a
head injury, although when present they may develop very
rapidly (even within the first hour) and carry a high mortality
rate. They are often associated with severe brain contusion and
it is this which makes them so potentially dangerous. Sometimes it becomes clear that a person has a subdural haematoma
weeks or months after a head injury which at the time may have
seemed trivial. Elderly people are particularly susceptible to
them. Symptoms of raised pressure in the head and brain distortion are delayed in these instances because bleeding is slow.

Brain swelling
Swelling of the brain may result from the release of certain
chemicals at the site of injury, in the same way that a finger
becomes swollen after trauma as a result of inflammation.

However, whereas elsewhere in the body the swelling itself usually causes no harm and subsides spontaneously, in the brain it adds to the already increased pressure within the skull. The resulting symptoms are similar to those from a blood clot, namely headache, sickness and eventually drowsiness. Sometimes the rise in pressure is transmitted to the back of the eyes and can be seen by a doctor using a tool called an ophthalmoscope. This is one of the reasons doctors will often be seen to shine a light in the eyes of patients who are under observation after a head injury.

A mild degree of brain swelling may go unnoticed. When it is severe it adds considerably to the patient's ill-health and may even put his or her life at risk. Raised pressure, whatever its cause, reduces the flow of blood through the vessels in the brain and the extraction of oxygen from the blood. It lessens the eventual degree of recovery of some patients because it interferes with the recovery of partly damaged areas of brain, which might have been salvaged if they had received a normal blood flow. This can be countered using various treatments, but it is best dealt with by prevention. A small probe can be inserted through a hole in the skull and connected to a pressure monitor. In this way the doctors can be alerted to an increase in the pressure before it becomes serious.

Brain swelling on just one side of the brain has its own problems. It causes the deep structures of the brain to be pushed across to the other side. More importantly, it distorts the brainstem, which becomes kinked or twisted and the nerves at the base of the brain could thus be damaged. Compression of the brainstem is a life-threatening condition.

Cerebrospinal fluid fistula
A cerebrospinal fluid (CSF) fistula is a fracture of the base of the skull which allows the fluid around the brain to leak out. If the front of the skull is affected, the fluid leaks into the throat or nose, whereas a leak from the ear points to a fracture of the middle part of the skull base. It may be blood-stained or clear, and it tastes salty. The discharge sometimes increases when leaning forward or with exertion. A CSF fistula may develop within the first few days after the head injury, or be delayed weeks or months. Many of them close up of their own accord, especially those resulting in a discharge from the ear, but others need

surgical treatment. If the leak is allowed to continue low pressure headaches may ensue, but the gravest risk is that of infection.

Meningitis

Germs may gain entry into the head following an injury either through an open fracture of the skull (especially through compound depressed fractures) or through a skull base fracture. In either case, the result is meningitis, which causes a high temperature, headache and neck stiffness. It is usually not difficult to recognise and treat, but there may be recurrences if the opening in the skull persists. It may be more difficult to deal with pockets of infection, called abscesses, within the substance of the brain.

Investigations

Many people with mild head injuries only require assessment from a doctor but others need radiological investigation. The decision whether to perform an X-ray or a brain scan depends on a number of factors, including whether or not the patient lost consciousness at the time of impact, whether there is a period of amnesia and whether he or she has any significant symptoms. If the answer to any of these questions is affirmative, or if there is scalp bruising, a skull X-ray will probably be done. The injured person may also undergo X-rays of the spine or other body parts, depending on the symptoms and the doctor's findings.

Skull X-ray

Like all the radiological procedures described in this chapter, X-rays are painless. Several pictures or views are usually taken with the purpose of ruling out or confirming the presence of a fracture. A fracture has implications for the long-term outlook as well as for treatment, since the risk of a blood clot developing in someone with an apparently mild head injury varies from one in seven thousand to one in eighty, depending on whether or not the skull has been fractured.

A fracture of the skull vault (its dome-shaped upper part) is usually readily recognisable on X-rays, but it may be confused with other markings on the skull, such as those from blood vessels, and so may be missed. Fractures of the base of the skull are often difficult to see on an X-ray because of the numerous natural irregularities in this region. If a doctor suspects that a fracture may be present, for instance, because there is deafness, bruising around the ear or a cerebrospinal fluid leak, a head scan will usually be carried out. Special views will be needed in the case of facial injuries to determine the presence and extent of fracturing of the bones around the eyes, cheekbones and jaw.

CT scan

A CT scan is much more informative than a standard X-ray because it shows the brain as well as the skull. Narrow beams of X-rays are aimed all the way around the head and the resulting images are processed by a computer (CT stands for computed tomography). In this way a number of 'slices' can be obtained from the top of the head down to the skull base. There is no discomfort to the patient and the radiation exposure is minimal. Sometimes the scan is repeated after the injection of a dye into a vein. Modern scanners are very fast and high quality images can often be obtained in a matter of minutes.

A scan is commonly performed if a person is drowsy after a head injury (especially if his or her conscious level is deteriorating) and if there are any signs of focal brain damage or of increased pressure in the brain. Sometimes this entails transferring the patient to another hospital, though naturally he or she will be closely supervised during the trip. Where a patient is seriously injured and in a deep coma it may be necessary to connect him or her to a ventilator before transfer to ensure that adequate breathing is maintained.

CT scans are generally better at picking up focal damage than diffuse low-level injury to the brain. They show cerebral contusion, haemorrhage and brain swelling, if present. They will also reveal a skull fracture, depressed fragments, foreign bodies and even the amount of soft tissue swelling. The appearances of a blood clot will vary depending on its age. There is a critical period at around two weeks after the head injury when it may be of the same appearance as the surrounding brain, making it difficult to recognise.

MR scan

Magnetic resonance (MR) scans are obtained by placing the subject in a powerful magnet. They do not employ X-rays and are very safe, but they cannot be used with people who have metal objects in the head (such as electronic implants or foreign bodies) because they might become dislodged and cause damage. Also, during the procedure it is more difficult to monitor closely a critically ill patient than with CT scanning. For this reason, as well as their high cost, MR scans are infrequently used with head-injured people despite the fact that they provide excellent images of the brain. They have a more clearly defined role in the assessment of brain damage once the immediate effects of the head injury have subsided.

Electroencephalography (EEG)

An electroencephalogram (EEG) is a record of the brain's electrical activity. It is obtained by attaching some wires to the scalp and is completely painless. It is different from X-rays and scans in that it reflects the function as opposed to the structure of the brain. Certain patterns of electrical activity are recognised as indicating concussion, particularly a general slowing of the waveforms. In practice, however, the diagnosis of concussion is usually made without resorting to an EEG. There are two circumstances in which an EEG may prove helpful, namely in the diagnosis of epilepsy and in the assessment of brain death. A patient may develop seizures as a consequence of a head injury, and it is useful to confirm that they are epileptic by recording an EEG. Typically, sharp waves appear, often in bursts. In other cases there may be no major fits but minor twitches of the face or hand may alert the doctor to the possibility of epilepsy and result in an EEG being carried out. (Epilepsy and its treatment is discussed further in the next chapter.) In the terminally ill patient who is completely unresponsive, an absence of any recordable brain waves on the EEG is a pointer to brain death.

Lumbar puncture

This consists of removing a sample of the fluid which bathes the brain (the cerebrospinal fluid) in order to analyse it in the laboratory. It is done by inserting a needle in the lower back after having deadened the skin with local anaesthetic. A lumbar puncture will never be carried out on a head-injured patient without having done a brain scan first. In fact, it is of little value in this setting except in those who are suspected of having meningitis. In such cases the fluid obtained from a lumbar puncture will show signs of infection.

Treatment

The treatment required immediately after a head injury will evidently vary from one person to another. The first step is an assessment of the head-injured person's condition, which starts at the scene of the accident. Paramedical and ambulance staff are trained to move an unconscious patient in such a way that further injury is avoided. Care of the airway is essential to allow normal breathing. Fractured limbs will be immobilised and an attempt made to stem any external bleeding by means of a pressure dressing.

Having arrived in hospital, the patient will be examined and a Glasgow or similar coma score will be obtained. If he or she is fully conscious and the coma score is high, treatment can be deferred. However, the patient will not be left unsupervised, as unforeseen deterioration can occur. Wounds will be dressed and stitched, if necessary. A decision will be made about whether a skull X-ray or CT scan is required. If there is no fracture, there are no abnormal findings when the person is examined by a doctor and he or she remains stable during a period of observation in the Accident and Emergency Department, they may well be allowed home with the instruction to return to hospital if there is any deterioration.

The position is quite different when the patient is drowsy or unconscious. His or her pulse and blood pressure will be checked to ensure that internal bleeding does not go unrecognised. A drip will be inserted into a vein to allow drugs to be injected and fluids to be delivered, if necessary. In patients with a Glasgow Coma Score of 8 or less a tube will be passed into the throat and he or she will be connected to a ventilator. This may require the use of drugs to sedate the patient, since restlessness increases the oxygen demand and leads to a rise in pressure in the head, quite apart from the distress the process causes. This initial evaluation and treatment takes only a few minutes but it ensures that the vital functions of breathing and circulation are safeguarded while other tests are carried out.

The next priority when a patient is unconscious is to establish whether there is a blood clot on the brain. A CT brain scan will usually be carried out promptly because a blood clot is present in about a third of severely head-injured patients. A pressure monitor may well be inserted through a small hole in the skull, which permits recording of the pressure inside the head. If it rises, the patient will usually have another brain scan, since it suggests that a blood clot, brain swelling or hydrocephalus is developing. Hydrocephalus is an enlargement of the cavities deep in the brain called the ventricles and is discussed in the next chapter.

If a clot is found it will require an operation if it is of substantial size and the patient's condition is deteriorating. Under a general anaesthetic a flap of skull bone is lifted to allow the clot to be removed and bleeding points identified and closed. The bone flap is then replaced. After the wound has fully healed small depressions may be left around the edge of the bone flap. There is a possibility of complications arising in the postoperative period caused by further haemorrhage or brain swelling. The patient will therefore be nursed in an intensive care or high dependency unit. Monitoring of the pressure inside the head and artificial breathing will be continued until his or her conscious level improves. In some cases it may be necessary to perform a tracheostomy, which is an opening in the windpipe through which a tube is passed: this is more likely to happen in severely injured patients who require support with breathing for more than a few days.

Whether or not surgery has been carried out, the nursing staff will keep a close eye on the patient's progress. Once out of danger, he or she will be nursed on a general surgical, orthopaedic or neurosurgical ward, depending on local circumstances and his or her other injuries. It is often necessary to use antibiotics and anticonvulsant drugs to ward off infection and fits respectively. Sometimes blood-thinning drugs (anticoagulants) are prescribed after the first few days to prevent blood clots forming in the leg veins while the injured person is immobile. Pressure stockings have the same function. As part of rehabilitation, the patient will then start to see occupational therapists, physiotherapists and speech therapists, as appropriate. Eventually he or she will be considered sufficiently fit to be discharged home, though often outside help will still be needed. The immediate crisis is over. The next stage is the process of recovery, aimed at overcoming or compensating for residual problems and aiding the injured person to become reintegrated into society.

3 Some physical effects of head injury

The post-traumatic syndrome

The terms post-traumatic syndrome (PTS) and post-concussional syndrome are used interchangeably to cover a wide range of symptoms experienced by people in the aftermath of a head injury, including headaches, dizziness, visual disturbance, nausea, fatigue, disordered sleep, irritability, forgetfulness, inability to concentrate and intolerance of alcohol. About fifty per cent of people have post-traumatic headaches after mild or moderate head injuries at work or in a road traffic accident. There has been much debate about the cause of PTS. Whereas some experts believe it to be due to a physical disturbance of brain function, others regard it as being primarily a psychological problem.

A number of interesting points have emerged from studies of the syndrome. PTS appears to occur only rarely in children or people who have suffered a sporting injury or a domestic accident. The symptoms of PTS are also generally more prominent in those who have had mild head injuries than in those with severe ones: arguably, the effects of a head injury should be proportional to its severity, and this is one of the reasons why some suggest that emotional factors are involved in causing the symptoms. The truth is that the condition is poorly understood and in all probability a number of factors are responsible for these complaints. On the one hand, concussion may cause mild disruption of the activity of the brain and changes in pressure inside the head could result in stretching of sensitive structures such as blood vessels or the layers surrounding the brain, the meninges. Having started as a physical condition, emotional factors may in some cases come into play and lead to a prolongation of the symptoms.

The outlook, or what doctors call the prognosis, of the post-traumatic syndrome is usually good. Often symptoms are quite troublesome during the first few weeks but after that they gradually improve. Full recovery may take anything between three months and two years. During this time it is best to remain active, though headaches and inability to concentrate are liable to interfere with sustained physical and mental effort. It is just as inadvisable for relatives or carers to be overprotective towards the sufferer as it is to dismiss his or her symptoms. When to return to work will depend very much on the circumstances of the individual case. If the only consequence of the accident has been a post-traumatic syndrome, that is, if there are no other major injuries, most people are able to go back to work within a few weeks, although in severe cases some months may elapse before normal full-time work is possible. Leisure pursuits and sports will often also have to be curtailed. The injured person may lack the confidence to drive for some time, though usually this effect is transient. It is important to realise that, although these symptoms may be very distressing, especially in the early stages after the head injury, full recovery is the norm.

Headache

A common and troublesome complaint after head injury is headache. Potential causes of headache following a mild head injury include muscle contraction, alterations in the blood supply to the brain, tenderness of the scalp and injury to the soft tissues of the neck. A serious cause such as an intracranial haemorrhage can usually be ruled out by an examination from a doctor who will look for some of the symptoms described in the previous chapter. The type of headache a person has varies to some extent depending on its cause. For instance, scarring of the scalp may result in a steady sensation of pressure at the site of impact, often combined with tenderness in the same area. If a small sensory nerve branch has been damaged there may also be tingling, or pins and needles, when the scalp is tapped.

Most commonly the headache takes the form of aching in a circumscribed area or in a band around the head. This type of pain probably arises in the muscles of the scalp and neck. A whiplash injury to the upper spine often accompanies head trauma, and in such cases there may be reflex contraction of neck muscles causing pain to spread to the head. Tension headaches occur on the same principle. Local stiffness and dizziness on moving the head may indicate the spinal origin of the headache. If there is pre-existing wear and tear in the joints of the neck, post-traumatic headaches can be quite persistent. When the accident has caused bruising of the face and around the eyes, strain on the eye muscles could be an additional source of pain. The best way of dealing with these headaches originating in the muscles of the face, neck and scalp is by taking simple pain-killers such as paracetamol.

Another type of headache consists of throbbing or pulsating pain which comes in waves and affects predominantly one side of the head. It is probably caused by stretching of the arteries of the scalp and neck, similar to that which occurs in migraine. This so-called post-traumatic migraine is not as common as muscle tension-type headaches following a head injury. There is sometimes a family history of migraine, or a history of previous headaches, perhaps forgotten, in the sufferer's youth. Nausea, flashing lights and sensitivity to noise often accompany the headache and force the sufferer to retire to bed in a darkened room. The same type of medication can effectively be used in post-traumatic as in standard migraine. Some drugs are designed to counter the attack once it has begun to develop. If headaches are frequent other drugs can be taken regularly as a preventive measure.

Inevitably, many people have more than one type of headache. There may be a combination of pain from local tissue damage, scalp or neck muscle contraction and changes in the blood supply to the brain. Emotional states such as fear of permanent damage and worry over employment may contribute to the headache. Depression can have the same effect. Difficulty sleeping, loss of appetite and despondency may set in, as well as the headaches. In these circumstances, doctors sometimes recommend an antidepressant drug. The sufferer should not feel that in accepting this advice he or she is 'giving in', since such treatment is likely to be short-lived, thus avoiding the risk of dependence.

Anosmia

Loss of the sense of smell is called anosmia. It may result either from a blocked nose or from damage to the nerves which carry information about smell to the brain. These nerves are called the olfactory nerves and are located underneath the front part of the brain. Anosmia is usually accompanied by loss of taste except for salty, bitter, sour and sweet tastes. These basic tastes are detected by the tongue, whereas we rely on smell to appreciate subtle aromas. Following a head injury anosmia develops in a proportion of people, probably because of bruising on the underside of the brain, or shearing of the olfactory nerves themselves. It usually affects both nostrils. The likelihood of losing the sense of smell depends to some extent on the severity of the head injury and its location. About one in twenty head-injured people attending hospital develop anosmia, though the figure increases to about one in four following severe injuries when the base of the skull has been fractured. Blows to the back of the head carry a higher risk of anosmia than do blows elsewhere. In some people partial damage to the olfactory nerves causes not loss but a distortion of smell, such that all odours appear to be the same. Sometimes this common odour is foul and unpleasant.

Anosmia not only reduces the enjoyment of food and drink, but it may put the sufferer at risk by not being able to detect smoke, gas or other toxic substances. There is no effective treatment other than prevention of danger, for example by installing smoke detectors. About a third of sufferers improve with the passage of time, mostly within the first six months after the head injury. Those with the mildest head injuries are more likely to recover.

Problems with hearing

Fractures of the skull base often damage the inner ear, usually on one side. This has consequences not only for hearing but also balance, since the inner ear contains organs concerned with both. The dizziness resulting from damage to the balance centre will be dealt with in the next section. As regards hearing, even in the unconscious patient deafness can be predicted if there are obvious signs of damage to the eardrum such as bleeding or a cerebrospinal fluid leak. Blood may accumulate on the inside of an intact eardrum, which can be detected by examining the ear with a special light called an otoscope. When the patient regains consciousness he or she may complain of deafness or tinnitus (an abnormal sound in the ear).

Hearing loss is a common consequence of skull fractures, but it may also occur with head trauma that does not result in any injury to the bones, in which case it is due to what is called inner ear concussion. Whereas deafness from a skull fracture can be quite profound, that from concussion tends to be mild. Sufferers complain of difficulty hearing conversation above a background noise, or their families or partners may say that they turn the television on too loud. A test of hearing (an audiogram) often shows the deafness to be worse where high-frequency sounds are concerned. In most cases, post-traumatic deafness improves in a matter of weeks without the need for treatment, especially in young people.

Tinnitus is an unpleasant symptom which troubles some patients who have suffered a closed head injury with inner ear damage. A whistling, ringing or roaring sound develops within days, though there may be a delay before the injured person reports it, especially if he or she is seriously ill. There is always some degree of hearing loss in the same ear. Tinnitus may be present all the time, but many people are only aware of it in a quiet environment, for instance, in bed at night. It is often more distressing and persistent than the associated hearing impairment.

Dizziness

Most often dizziness after a head injury is a manifestation of a post-traumatic syndrome which includes headaches, mental fatigue and/or irritability. As pointed out earlier, this is usually a temporary phenomenon which is rarely disabling. Some people complain of light-headedness and darkening of vision on sitting up or getting out of bed. Such symptoms are due to slow adjustment of their blood pressure to changes in posture. These problems are short-lived and require no action other than advice to get up more slowly. Other people notice a feeling of faintness when they look up. This occurs most often in the elderly, whose arteries are less flexible and may become kinked when the neck is extended, thus reducing the blood flow to the brain. Here, too, it is sensible to avoid the movement which brings on the symptoms.

A more troublesome symptom after a head injury is that of vertigo. This is a feeling of giddiness or swaying, often on movement, associated with nausea and loss of balance when standing. The doctor may also notice a characteristic wobbliness of the eyes called nystagmus. This combination of symptoms points to an injury to the labyrinth (the organ in the inner ear devoted to balance), though brainstem damage may have similar effects. When X-rays do not reveal signs of a skull base fracture, it is assumed that the injured person is suffering from labyrinthine concussion. At times the vertigo only occurs when a person assumes a certain position and it is then called positional vertigo. Like cerebral concussion, labyrinthine concussion is a temporary problem which improves within weeks. The attacks of vertigo become less severe and the intervals between them lengthen, though complete resolution of the problem can take two or three years. The sufferer may develop understandable fear of heights which persists even after the tendency to vertigo has subsided. It is usually possible to suppress the symptoms with drugs similar to those used against seasickness until natural recovery takes place.

Post-traumatic epilepsy

Epilepsy is a tendency to recurrent attacks of altered consciousness due to disturbed electrical activity in the brain. This definition encompasses two essential elements, namely that there must be more than one attack and that the disturbance is electrical. A single fit does not constitute epilepsy, nor do recurrent faints. There is much fear surrounding the diagnosis of epilepsy and it is therefore important for the sufferer to understand what it means. Epilepsy is not a mental illness but rather a transient disturbance of the activity of the brain. Some patients develop it in childhood due to a constitutional predisposition (that is, they inherit it) while in others it results from a stroke, brain tumour, head injury or exposure to certain toxic substances (including excessive alcohol intake). In some cases a dormant predisposition to epilepsy may become manifest after head trauma.

People who suffer from epilepsy have fits or seizures, with periods of normal health in between. These fits may be minor or major, depending on whether or not consciousness is completely lost. A minor attack may take the form of an absence, focal twitching or a so-called complex partial seizure. An 'absence' consists of staring into space for a few seconds. A focal fit is one where there is twitching of a foot or hand which then spreads up the limb. A complex partial seizure, as its name implies, is a combination of various bodily sensations (an odd smell, butterflies in the stomach), psychological features (such as out of body experiences) and what are called motor automatisms (twitching or fidgeting). Major seizures are readily recognisable, for they cause a sudden loss of consciousness, stiffening of the body and jerking of the limbs. Such a convulsion may last three to four minutes and usually leaves the person feeling drained for several hours. All of these types of seizures may occur after trauma to the head, except absences which invariably start in childhood.

Whether or not someone who has suffered head trauma develops epilepsy depends on numerous factors, amongst which the most important is the severity of the injury. If there has been neither loss of consciousness nor any post-traumatic amnesia, there is no likelihood of epilepsy. At the other extreme, someone who has been unconscious with a depressed skull fracture runs a risk of developing epilepsy of about fifty per cent. This is because the fragments of bone at the fracture site are liable to damage the surface of the brain, leaving a scar which can then cause fits. When there is a skull fracture without the bones being pushed towards the brain, then the risk of epilepsy is minimal. Another likely cause of fits is the presence of a blood clot in the brain or on its surface.

The timing of the seizures is also important. Fits occurring in the first week after the injury are called early epilepsy. Many of these are focal fits or major seizures with a focal onset. They often prompt the doctors to do a brain scan, if one had not already been done, because they may be a pointer to bleeding in the brain which requires surgery. Seizures in the first week increase the risk of the late development of post-traumatic epilepsy.

While these details may appear rather frightening, it should be remembered that only a small minority of people have a depressed skull fracture, early seizures or a brain clot. For those who have had a head injury leading to unconsciousness or post-traumatic amnesia but without any of these complications, the chances that they will ever have any fits as a consequence of their head injury are only one to two per cent. The risk halves in the first year and continues to drop after that, until it becomes negligible by about five years after the accident. These estimates apply to non-missile head injuries only: the risks of epilepsy following a bullet wound to the head are altogether higher.

If a person develops seizures it is likely he or she will be treated with anticonvulsant drugs. Indeed, it is possible that such drugs will be prescribed for prevention of seizures, even when a fit has not actually occurred. There are a wide variety of such drugs available and they are usually very effective. Often it is possible to stop the drugs after two to three years without the fits recurring. Epilepsy is eminently treatable and normally places no major restrictions on the sufferer except that he or she will not be allowed to drive for a year from the date of the last fit, and working with heavy machinery or at heights should be avoided during the same period. HGV and PSV drivers will lose their licences. In other respects the sufferer should lead a normal life, secure in the knowledge that the more time goes by the less likely it is that further fits will occur.

When anticonvulsant drugs are prescribed, there are sometimes unwanted side-effects. Such drugs act on the brain and it is therefore very common for them to cause some drowsiness or tiredness. To some extent this depends on the dose, so unless it is a matter of urgency because fits are occurring frequently, the doctor will usually start by prescribing a small amount which is gradually increased until a suitable dose for the person's weight and age is reached. In children some drugs can cause restlessness or difficulty concentrating, a change which is often first noticed by their teachers. There may also be problems with reduced alertness in adults but they tend to be less important than in a child or adolescent faced with all manner of new challenges at school. This is the reason why doctors usually try to withdraw anticonvulsant drugs after a year or two if there have been no further fits.

Some drugs are liable to cause indigestion or rashes similar to those resulting from an allergic reaction. This is not usually a problem, since there are many kinds of anticonvulsant drugs and it is nearly always possible to find one which suits each individual person. Anaemia, some disturbance of the liver and changes in the hair may also occur in a small number of cases, particularly when the older anticonvulsant drugs are used. All of these can be detected by a doctor and put right. In other cases symptoms such as confusion and unsteadiness may arise when the sufferer has inadvertently been given too high a dose. This, too, can be corrected by doing a blood test and reducing the dose accordingly. None of these effects are permanent and in most cases the benefits of being free of fits greatly outweigh the inconvenience of side-effects which may develop. Lastly, it is worth pointing out that women on anticonvulsant medication should consult their doctors before considering becoming pregnant.

Hydrocephalus

Most of the consequences of a head injury dealt with above improve with the passage of time. When there is worsening of the patient's condition in the months which follow the accident, this may be due either to the unmasking of a pre-existing disorder or to the development of a delayed complication. For instance, increasing headaches and confusion may signal a gradually expanding chronic blood clot. Equally, progressive mental deterioration after a head injury may be due to hydrocephalus. It is worth stressing that both of these complications are rare. Hydrocephalus is an enlargement of the cavities deep in the brain called the ventricles. These cavities contain cerebrospinal fluid which flows onto the surface of the brain and protects it. After a head injury there is sometimes poor absorption of this fluid, causing it to accumulate steadily in the ventricles. As it does so the brain becomes increasingly compressed and the sufferer's condition deteriorates. He or she may become apathetic and confused. Headaches develop or existing headaches worsen, sometimes with associated sickness. In more advanced cases there may be incontinence, disturbances of vision and unsteadiness of gait. Examination by a doctor will show signs of raised pressure inside the head and the diagnosis is confirmed by performing a brain scan. If the hydrocephalus is mild or the patient is frail, the doctors will sometimes decide to do nothing other than keep him or her under observation. If the condition is more serious surgery will be carried out to drain the excess fluid away from the brain to either the heart or the abdomen through a tube called a shunt. The majority of patients who have had a shunt improve, though the operation is not free of risk, particularly for the elderly.

Balance and co-ordination

Limb movements may be disturbed for one of two reasons: the limb is weak or it lacks co-ordination. Weakness down one side of the body is called a hemiparesis and may occur after an injury to the opposite side of the brain, more specifically to the frontal lobe. The affected limbs tend to be stiff as well; this is called spasticity. The arm or the leg may be more severely affected, depending on where precisely the damage occurred. In some people who have suffered widespread brain damage both arms and legs are affected. They walk stiffly and have difficulty using their hands for simple day-to-day tasks. In the most serious cases they may be virtually helpless, unable to stand or walk and dependent on others for washing, dressing, toileting and feeding. Such severely disabled people require a great deal of care and supervision. Because the muscles are stiff they will need to be stretched at regular intervals, since otherwise there is a risk that they will become permanently shortened (this condition is called contractures). When the weakness is only partial the sufferer may well be able to perform the necessary stretching movements or at least contribute to them. In other cases a physiotherapist or, after training, a relative will perform stretching exercises to loosen the affected limbs. This ensures that when strength eventually returns to the limb movements will not be hindered by muscle contractures.

Some people have difficulty using their limbs not because they are weak but because they are clumsy. Trembling and loss of dexterity of the hands, difficulty judging distances, slurring of speech and unsteadiness of gait are all features of what is called a cerebellar syndrome. The cerebellum is located at the back of the brain and deals with co-ordination of all voluntary movements. When it is damaged it is no longer possible to move smoothly because the various muscles are not acting in synchrony, even though their strength is normal. A multidisciplinary approach is needed to rehabilitate people with this problem, involving physiotherapists, occupational therapists and specialist nurses.

Incontinence

Incontinence means the inability to control one's bladder and/or bowels. Used without qualification it usually means urinary incontinence which is much commoner than loss of bowel control. In the early stages after a severe head injury the unconscious person is unaware of bodily functions and the nursing staff will be alert to the possibility of either incontinence or retention of urine. A catheter (a small flexible tube) is often used to drain the urine and is kept in the bladder until the person's level of consciousness improves. The risk of this procedure is that germs may gain entry into the bladder and cause an infection called cystitis. In order to avoid this, specimens of urine are sent to the laboratory for testing at frequent intervals, and if any infection is detected appropriate treatment is started.

The great majority of people who are incontinent in the early stages after a head injury regain control of their bladder. In those who have suffered severe brain damage this is not always the case. The sufferer may be left with both a diminished perception of bladder fullness and a diminished ability to empty his or her bladder. Nevertheless, as sensation and control are usually reduced rather than lost, bladder retraining can often be achieved. This is done by encouraging the sufferer to empty the bladder regularly, if necessary by stroking trigger areas such as the lower abdomen or inner thigh. Drinks should be avoided late at night to reduce the likelihood of incontinence. A bottle or commode is sometimes provided by the social services if there is difficulty getting to the toilet. When there is continuous dribbling of urine in male sufferers a condom sheath may be applied, which drains into a collection bag attached to the leg. This is especially useful to keep the person dry at night or when going out. Lastly, intermittent catheterisation is sometimes advised when the bladder does not empty properly despite all attempts at retraining. This involves passing a small tube which is then withdrawn after all the urine has drained off. It should be emphasised, however, that long-term incontinence is rare, even if the head injury was severe.

Persistent vegetative state

Someone who is unconscious is said to be in a coma. When the coma is prolonged this is associated with brain damage, though it does not necessarily mean that some degree of recovery is impossible. For instance, many adult patients who have been in a coma for one week after a head injury will return to a satisfying personal and social life. There is, however, a small group of people whose injuries have been so profound and extensive that they remain in a coma. Indeed, if the brainstem has ceased to function the patient is unable to breathe and can only survive by remaining attached to a ventilator. When there is total absence of movement and spontaneous breathing and no response to a variety of cranial nerve reflexes, the patient is said to be brain dead. There is no prospect of recovery and life-support systems will therefore be turned off. Relatives may be asked for permission to obtain organs for transplantation.

People who have been in a prolonged coma and show no signs of recovery but nevertheless can breathe on their own are not brain dead, since at least one brainstem function is maintained (that of breathing). Such patients are said to be in a persistent vegetative state (PVS). This term is not applied to patients who have recently been rendered unconscious, however deeply, since as pointed out before the great majority will improve, but only to those who, despite all medical care, remain unresponsive for weeks or months. The longer the coma, the less likely it is that meaningful improvement will occur. Such patients may make unintelligible sounds, open their eyes or move briefly. They can feel pain and react in a reflex manner to sound and touch. However, they cannot for the most part hear, see, move purposefully or think in the accepted sense. Their limbs are held stiffly and often contractures (shortening of the muscles) develop. They have no control over their bowels and bladder. They need to be fed, usually by means of a tube passed into their stomach. The care of such patients raises a number of difficult ethical issues beyond the scope of this book.

Helping recovery from coma and PVS

During a coma the person may vary between being quite still and unresponsive, and becoming more active and opening his or her eyes. Comas can vary in depth and the patient may seem more active at some times than others. Occasionally it can be difficult for the medical staff to pinpoint precisely when it has ended. Understandably relatives find coma extremely stressful, because it may not always be possible for the doctors to say with certainty what the person's chances of survival are and they may fear for the condition he or she will be in at the end of the coma. Many relatives invest a good deal of effort talking to the patient and bring along familiar objects for him or her to touch, or tape recorded messages from friends. It is not really clear how effective this is in shortening the coma, although there are anecdotal accounts that it can help and many relatives are confident that their efforts make a difference. In recent years a body of research has developed into what are called Coma Arousal or Stimulation Therapies for people who are unconscious or in a persistent vegetative state. The nature of these treatments tends to vary considerably, but in essence they consist of a programme in which the person's senses (that is, vision, hearing, touch, smell and taste) are systematically stimulated for varying periods in the expectation that this will assist in lightening the coma or PVS. Relatives often play an important role in helping staff and, for example, may bring along favourite music to play to the person. Sometimes the entire treatment is administered by the family. Some research studies have suggested that these treatments shorten coma, although there is much debate about whether this really is so, and whether stimulation influences the long-term outcome. At the moment it is not clear how useful such treatment is. Certainly there is no reason to think that stimulation does any harm and at worst it may have no effect at all; in the circumstances, many relatives prefer to give this approach a try, rather than do nothing.

Dos and don'ts

What a person should or should not do after a head injury will, of course, depend a great deal on what, if any, handicaps may be present. Sufferers and carers often wonder how safe it is for someone who has had a head injury to go out, play sports or pursue a hobby. The general rule is that common sense should prevail. Initially alcohol should not be drunk at all, or only in small amounts. Heavy exercise may not be well tolerated for some time after a head injury, causing both tiredness and headaches, but a gradual build-up of physical activity will for most people slowly overcome these problems. Contact sports should be avoided until all symptoms have subsided. A man who has had surgery on the brain will be told by his doctors that he should not play rugby or competitive football again. The dents or depressions on the skull which result from surgery need not be a cause for concern when undertaking normal day-to-day activities, since the brain remains well protected, but they might represent points of weakness if a person attempts to head a ball. Other pursuits such as swimming, fishing, playing golf or going for walks are entirely appropriate and are all invaluable in promoting a gradual return to normality.

4 Thinking and reasoning: cognitive problems

Head injury, even if not severe, may affect what are called our cognitive abilities. Cognitive is a general term used to refer to thinking skills such as memory and attention, the ability to reason logically and to understand and produce speech. In the following pages we will look at some of the most common cognitive problems after head injury and how they can either be overcome or circumvented using simple techniques. Not everyone who has a head injury later suffers from these problems and those who do vary enormously in the extent to which they are affected: some are rendered quite dependent because of the psychological changes they have undergone, while others are able to lead essentially normal lives. For some people the main problem is forgetfulness, whereas others have additional difficulties, such as in speaking or thinking coherently. They may also have undergone some of the personality changes that are discussed in the next chapter. The precise pattern of difficulties varies according to a number of factors, most particularly the severity and precise site of the brain damage: a severe head injury which has a widespread effect on the brain is, as one might expect, more likely to result in lasting and widespread cognitive problems; whereas relatively discreet damage, perhaps affecting a localised area of the brain, may leave many faculties intact and result in relatively circumscribed cognitive problems.

Problems with memory

Perhaps the most common cognitive problem after head injury is forgetfulness, which can range from minor forgetfulness where the person has difficulty remembering day-to-day details such as items of shopping or telephone numbers, through to severe and disabling conditions when he or she cannot recall conversations from one hour to the next and is unable to live independently.

Christine

Christine was involved in a car crash in which she was knocked unconscious for over an hour. When she came to, she was dazed and confused for more than a day. Nevertheless, apart from cuts and bruises and a broken leg, there were no serious physical injuries and she soon made a good medical recovery. A few months after leaving hospital she went back to her job as a cashier in a bank. At first Christine's employers were under-standing and encouraged her to pace herself and did not push her. After a few weeks, however, she was expected to work at her usual speed and had to remember transactions, details of customers' accounts and so on. Christine soon noticed that her memory was not as sharp as it had been, and unless she made a particular effort she forgot customers' details and tasks she had been asked to do. She found that she had to keep lists to make sure she did not overlook details and if she did not write things down straight away she tended to forget them. At home she had similar problems, although as she was under less pressure there they were less worrying. When she watched soap operas on television, she had difficulty remembering the story-line from previous episodes, although eventually it came back to her. When she went shopping she would forget at least one of the things she had gone for, so she took to writing everything down. Her family soon noticed that she was more forgetful, and her memory became something of a family joke.

Christine's case is a common one in that, although she appeared to have made a good, if not complete, physical recovery, she had nevertheless suffered damage to her memory, which although not serious was frustrating. She was fortunate that to a large extent she was able to cover up the problem at work and prevent it from affecting her performance. Minor forgetfulness like Christine's may not be significant in many jobs and can easily be tolerated or overlooked, but for a pilot or a surgeon, such problems may signal the end of that person's career.

Paul

Paul, a builder, suffered a severe head injury when he fell from a roof while erecting scaffolding. He was in a coma for several days, and afterwards suffered from muscle weakness affecting both his left leg and arm. As a result he had great difficulty getting in and out of bed and chairs. He could only walk for short distances, and then only with the support of his wife Anne. According to Anne, however, his most serious problem did not lie in his physical limitations, but in his forgetfulness, and it was this which caused her the most stress. Paul could not remember when he and Anne married, and he had only a vague recollection of his past jobs. Almost every day he would repeat remarks five or six times, or ask Anne a question and then repeat it within the hour. If, for instance, they were due to go to the clinic, Anne would tell him what time they were leaving, but within what seemed like moments he would cheerfully ask again when they were due to set off, without showing any signs of remembering what Anne had said previously, or any concern at her exasperation. Each time she dutifully answered but without fail he would repeat the question. The stress of Paul's forgetfulness on Anne was enormous and she was often at her wits' end trying to cope with his repeated questions.

Paul's forgetfulness was clearly of a different order from Christine's, although it is nevertheless typical of a severely head-injured person. Part of the problem with Paul's memory was that it was not a problem for him. He was unable to recall that he had forgotten things, and consequently made no effort to overcome his forgetfulness, but simply enquired, as anyone would, if something slipped his mind. After serious head injuries, the main victim is often not the head-injured person, but rather the relatives (in this case Anne), who have to cope with never-ending questions. Anne was also typical of many relatives in that her main concern about the way Paul had changed was not the fact that she had to help him with chores such as washing and toileting, but rather the stress caused by his forgetfulness and repetitiveness.

What then are the main kinds of memory problems that occur after head injury? There are three main types: retrograde mnesia, post-traumatic amnesia and short-term memory problems.

Retrograde amnesia
Many people have difficulty remembering events that happened before their injury. If they were involved in a car crash they may, for example, remember setting out on the journey but

then nothing else before the accident. This period is called retrograde amnesia, which means that there is a period of forgetfulness, or amnesia, for events before the injury. This interval is usually of only a few minutes' duration, but sometimes people cannot remember what happened for days or even weeks beforehand, or if they can remember at all their recall is patchy and hazy. Retrograde amnesia usually covers the longest period of time immediately after the injury; as time passes gaps in memory are filled until the forgotten period stablises as covering particular moments and this does not subsequently change. Very commonly the moment of impact itself is not remembered and, in fact, if someone can remember what happened to them it is unlikely that he or she has sustained a head injury of any severity. It is sometimes assumed that a person is unable to remember what happened at the time of the injury because he or she unconsciously wants to forget the trauma. In most cases, however, this is unlikely to be the explanation, and the forgetfulness is due to the disruption to the brain which interferes with memories being stored.

Post-traumatic amnesia

Whether or not a person has been in a coma there is usually a period after a head injury when they are somewhat confused and do not appear to be taking things in. They may also be disoriented, that is, they do not know the date or what day or year it is, or even with certainty where they are. Alternatively they may seem to take things in, but it later transpires that their working memory is not functioning properly and they forget things from one moment to the next. This state is called post-traumatic amnesia, and can last for only a minute or two or up to several months before clearing. Post-traumatic amnesia is important because it is a useful index of the severity of the head injury and the likely extent of diffuse brain damage. A short interval of post-traumatic amnesia in the order of minutes or an hour means that any damage to the brain is likely to have been mild. However, if the interval of amnesia extends to a day or a week or more, the greater is the degree of diffuse damage to the brain. Lengthy post-traumatic amnesia means an increased likelihood of subsequent psychological problems such as memory and personality difficulties. This is not always the case, however, and some people who experience long periods of amnesia have relatively few problems, whereas others with mild or moderate injuries later have significant difficulties.

Short-term memory problems

When the period of post-traumatic amnesia has passed and the head-injured survivor is medically well, or at least stable, it is possible to see whether he or she has suffered any enduring memory problems. These problems vary considerably, but, in a typical case, memory for day-to-day matters such as recalling telephone numbers, messages, or what has happened in a television programme, is affected. This indicates that the person has suffered damage to his or her short-term memory. It should be said that the term short-term memory is used to refer to a variety of different processes by different professionals, and for psychologists who study how memory works it can have a quite specific and technical meaning. However, such technicalities are of little importance to sufferers and their relatives, and it is quite acceptable to use the term loosely to refer to problems with learning and retaining new information. In contrast, events or details from many years ago, such as the name of an old schoolfriend or a childhood holiday, may be remembered quite well, even though one might expect that these memories would be harder to recall. Sufferers are often aware of this anomaly and remark on it, and relatives are sometimes puzzled by the apparent discrepancy. Christine, whose memory problems were described earlier, suffered from mild short-term memory problems, whereas Paul had a profound, if not total, short-term memory failure, as well as difficulty recalling events from the distant past.

The type and severity of memory problems depends on a number of factors. Damage to different areas of the brain may, for example, result in different kinds of memory problems. This is because not all memories are stored in the same areas of the brain. Memories for written material, such as newspaper articles, or for conversations, are usually stored in the left side of the brain (called the left hemisphere), whereas memories for faces or music are stored in the right side (the right hemisphere). If in the course of an injury the left side of the brain, say, has borne the brunt of any damage, it is possible later to have a satisfactory memory for faces but poor recall for conversations or novels. Likewise, damage to the right side of the brain may have the opposite effect. Certain emotional states can have an impact and influence memory. Strong feelings of depression or anxiety can undermine memory because they interfere with a person's concentration and so affect the ability to take in information. Unlike memory problems resulting from damage to the brain, forgetfulness due to emotional problems is potentially reversible, and when the depression or anxiety is treated, perhaps by medication or counselling, memory is likely to improve.

Memory problems can be quite variable, and sufferers may forget some details but have no difficulty remembering something else quite similar. Relatives can find these apparent inconsistencies extremely frustrating and think they are due to lack of effort, and that with more application the head-injured person could improve his or her recall. There is no doubt that lack of effort may be an important factor in some cases, although it should be borne in mind that this in itself may be part of a change in character due to brain damage. On the other hand, some people do play on their otherwise real forgetfulness, and it is not uncommon to hear relatives wrily complain that whereas the head-injured person forgets to tidy up, he or she has no difficulty remembering when a favourite television programme is scheduled!

Difficulty concentrating

Brain damage may affect the ability to concentrate on books, conversations or studies. As with forgetfulness, the severity of the problem ranges from people who experience only occasional and subtle difficulties, perhaps mainly when they are fatigued, through to those who cannot even attempt to read because they are so distractible and lacking in patience. Attention involves a number of different processes, such as the ability to attend for long periods, ignoring distractions, and being able to focus on more than one thing at a time; and any or all of these different abilities may be impaired after brain damage.

Sustained attention

'My mind wanders when I try to read a book'

After head injury some people have difficulty with what is called sustained attention, that is, in concentrating for prolonged periods on the same thing, such as the television or their studies. People with this problem may find that when they read they tire easily, their mind drifts off what they are reading and they end up thinking about something else. Many jobs have monotonous aspects, such as checking records, supervising machinery, and working out figures, and it is when dealing with such tasks that problems may emerge. The difficulty is not necessarily that the head-injured person has lost the ability to do the task, but rather that he or she is simply unable to work at it over a lengthy period. One way around the problem is to reorganise one's approach and work for short periods followed by rests. A student, for instance, might change his or her work habits so that instead of studying intensively for long hours close to the exams, he or she completes just an hour's work every evening. By doing a little work often, it may be possible to avoid over-taxing oneself. Although the problem may not be cured it can sometimes be circumvented.

Selective attention

'I can't concentrate on my studies if there are noises in the house'

Many tasks such as reading or homework have to be done against a background of noise or other distractions which we usually 'filter out' automatically, without difficulty. In other words, we select what we will pay attention to and ignore irrelevant events or details. However, after brain trauma this ability to attend selectively can be impaired, and a person may be easily distracted and have difficulty tolerating noise, and prefer quiet environments. Sometimes the distractibility can be quite severe; one head-injured man, while being asked by his doctor about his problems, glanced around the room looking at the medical equipment, peered out of the window, and commented on noises in the corridor outside which the doctor had not himself noticed. He had a severe problem with selective attention: he was unable to filter out and ignore irrelevant distractions and was continually drawn to whatever happened to impinge upon him. Few people who have had a head injury are quite so distractible, and indeed for many the problems they experience are quite subtle. It may be primarily in noisy environments like a pub that they have problems keeping track of a conversation, or in a busy shop they have difficulty reckoning change, whereas otherwise they do not experience significant difficulties.

Divided attention

'I can't listen to what the teacher is saying and take notes at the same time'

This remark was made by a college student who had impaired divided attention: that is, he had difficulty paying attention to two things at the same time. Having to cope with two or more tasks simultaneously may make the head-injured person feel overwhelmed, so that he or she soon gives up. This can be extremely disabling, since it is not uncommon that we have to cope with competing demands. At work, for instance, it may be necessary to juggle tasks such as talking on the phone and taking notes, or operating machinery while talking to a colleague.

Attentional problems are common after head injury although they can initially be overlooked by hospital staff and relatives who may focus on overcoming more obvious problems to do with mobility or toileting. During recuperation there are also usually relatively few intellectual demands that would highlight such difficulties, and it may not be until some time has passed and the survivor tries to get back to work, where he or she is expected to be as competent and alert as the next person, that problems become obvious. Poor concentration can be as disabling as a physical handicap, if not more so, and is often one of the main reasons why people who have had relatively mild injuries nevertheless find themselves unable to hold down a job.

Producing and understanding language

In most right-handed people the left side of the brain (left hemisphere) is the part of the brain responsible for understanding and producing language. In left-handed people the brain is organised slightly differently, and the right side of the brain (right hemisphere) may also have a role to play in language. If the language centres of the brain are damaged, the head-injured person will suffer from what is called aphasia. **Aphasia** is the term given to a partial or complete loss of the ability to produce speech or understand what is said. Since most people are right-handed, and their left hemisphere is responsible for language, aphasia is usually a sign that the left side of the brain has been damaged.

For some people the main problem is that they are unable to produce speech. They pick the wrong word or choose nonsensical words, and, with difficulty, produce brief, fragmented sentences. However, while their speech is not normal, their understanding of what is said may be quite adequate, and by pointing or making signs they can show they understand what is said to them. Others have problems with both comprehension and speech production. The reason for this is that the area of the brain responsible for understanding speech is not the same as that responsible for producing speech. As a result it is possible to have difficulty with speech production but not comprehension. If the comprehension area is damaged, however, this inevitably has an impact on the person's ability to speak sensibly. Aphasia should be distinguished from what is called dysarthria. **Dysarthria** is when the areas of the brain which control the muscles involved in producing speech are damaged. If this happens speech is slurred, hesitant and slow. People with aphasia often suffer from a degree of dysarthria, and the combination of aphasia and dysarthria can cause their speech to be difficult and sometimes impossible to understand.

After head injury most people do not, in fact, suffer a serious breakdown in their use of language, and aphasia is relatively uncommon. However, this is not to say that there are no problems and there may be subtle difficulties. A common problem is **anomia**, which means difficulty in finding the right word. People who suffer from anomia talk and understand normally, but every now and then they get stuck for words or they cannot retrieve a person's name. This is a problem with which we are all familiar to some degree and most of us experience 'tip of the tongue' difficulties from time to time. After a head injury, however, the problem can be severe or crop up much more frequently. To get around it some people keep talking while they try to remember the word, or they describe what they are referring to. A further problem is difficulty in keeping track of a conversation in which several people are contributing. Some head-injured people cope well talking one-to-one, but when they have to keep up in a group conversation, they tend to drop out. The problem is that they are slow at processing what is said and forming an answer. In other words, they are capable of under-standing and producing speech, but the rate at which they operate has slowed down. This may be due to poor attention, as talking in a group is a good example of having to take in information quickly from several different sources, monitor people's reactions, and time one's intervention: in other words selective, sustained and divided attention are all needed, and if these are impaired it may be difficult to keep up.

Problem-solving skills

Head injury can affect how flexibly a person solves problems, plans, organises and co-ordinates his or her behaviour, and therefore how productive they are and how easily they attain goals. These abilities are usually controlled by the frontal lobes, which are the areas of the brain behind the forehead. Research studies have established that the frontal lobes are extremely important in maintaining self-control, so that we do not act impulsively but plan and regulate our actions. Because of their location, however, these parts of the brain are a common site of injury, and this may mean that a person with a brain trauma is impulsive, lacks self-restraint and acts without thought for the future. They may be unable to reflect on what they are doing, or more particularly what they are not doing or doing wrong, and consequently make repeated mistakes. They may take things literally because they find it hard to think in abstract terms. Sometimes they have the skills to work or study but neverthe-less find it hard to co-ordinate them effectively.

Mark

Before his head injury Mark was a college student completing a computer course. He was bright and highly successful and usually achieved good grades. After his head injury he did not return to college immediately, although this remained his aim. His father said that Mark sat every day in his bedroom at his home computer and apparently worked diligently at programmes to get himself back to his old standard. He worked most days for a few hours and frequently talked about his work and read computer magazines. However, as the months went by his father began to notice that none of this activity seemed to lead anywhere or be productive. The father also noticed that in other areas Mark had difficulty completing tasks and was easily muddled. On one occasion he tried to help his father strip down and clean a motorbike, a task he had done many times before his injury. However, he got confused as to how to go about it and which tools to use, and he put the components back together in the wrong order and then had to dismantle parts of it again to correct what he had done. He tried to reassemble the bike in the same incorrect manner several times, despite being aware that he was doing it wrong. As a result he became extremely frustrated, threw down his tools and gave up.

Mark's problem was that although he knew from past experience how to dismantle the bike, he had difficulty planning how to set about the work and consequently became confused and frustrated. Head injury can cause people to become quite rigid and inflexible. When dealing with problems they may take a particular approach, and if this does not work out they have difficulty adapting and thinking of another. As a result they keep trying the same failed strategy over again and repeat the same mistakes: this is called 'perseveration', which means that the person perseveres with a strategy even when it is incorrect and is unable to learn from experience. When Mark tried unsuccessfully to rebuild the engine he could not stop to work out an alternative strategy but simply dismantled the pieces and started again. Sometimes people perseverate when speaking and, for example, they repeat stock phrases or remarks in a repetitive manner. Repetitive remarks can be extremely difficult for carers and relatives to bear and understandably tax their patience.

Loss of insight

Many people are all too aware of the fact that they have changed after a head injury, and are distressed by their cognitive and physical disabilities. Understandably this awareness can cause despondency and depression which in turn can lead to further problems. However, some head-injured people have little or no awareness of their limitations and when asked will deny that there is anything wrong, whereas their relatives say that they are greatly changed.

Alexander

Alexander suffered a severe head injury when he was knocked off his motorbike on the way to work one morning. He had neurosurgery to remove a blood clot from his brain and was in a coma for several days. When he went to hospital for a check-up a year after the accident, his wife said that he was extremely forgetful and repeatedly asked questions and forgot her answers. His train of thought was slow and he wandered from one topic to the next with only the loosest connection between them. It was common for him to start talking about one thing and within moments drift on to another unrelated topic. When asked whether he was having any problems, however, Alexander said that his only complaint was that he could not lift his arm to shave, and when specifically asked about his memory he replied that it was fine. The doctor at the clinic noticed that he had problems finding words, and on several occasions during their discussion he came to a complete halt because he could not find the right word. When asked if he had any problems remembering words, however, Alexander replied that his speech was fine and he appeared oblivious of the problems he had exhibited only moments before.

Michael

Michael suffered a serious head injury when he came off his bike in a bicycle race. Afterwards he was much changed and his mother, with whom he lived, said that he was distractible, could not sit still and always seemed edgy and 'hyped up'. On several occasions he went to the shops and came back with the wrong item, and could not be relied upon to pass on messages. On a number of occasions he lit the cooker to heat food and then went into the lounge to watch television and forgot all about the cooking. Each time a disaster was only averted when his mother smelt burning. She tried to get him to keep a daily list to overcome his forgetfulness, and every morning she made a point of reminding him of things that had to be done that day. However, Michael himself had no complaints about his memory and he ignored all these strategies. When pressed, he vaguely admitted that he was perhaps a little forgetful, but he said it was not a serious problem and he thought he could easily overcome it with effort.

It is not uncommon for the views of a head-injured person and their relatives to differ considerably. They may agree about the presence of physical complaints such as difficulty in walking or visual problems, but disagree about psychological problems such as forgetfulness or slowness and personality changes. On the whole, relatives tend to be much more aware of the psychological effects of the injury. Loss of insight is a consequence of the damage to the brain and, to some extent, may protect the head-injured person from becoming distressed and developing depression, for which his or her family may be grateful. On the other hand, attempts to overcome problems are likely to be difficult, as the sufferer is unlikely to make much effort in rehabilitation if they do not consider there is anything wrong. Loss of insight may also mean that a head-injured person represents a danger both to themselves and to others - for example, they might use electrical or gas appliances and forget about them, so causing a fire. Relatives should be on their guard against such eventualities and ensure that they and the head-injured person are not unwittingly put at risk. Some head-injured people also have difficulty coping with money and spend recklessly, regardless of their real needs or whether they are getting into debt. They may also be vulnerable to exploitation from people who are prepared to take advantage of them. Once again relatives have to be alert to these potential problems and may need to take steps to ensure that money is not spent unwisely. If someone is unable to manage their finances, perhaps because of lack of judgement or extreme forgetfulness, then it may be necessary for the Court of Protection to step in and take charge of their affairs. This happens on the recommendation of a doctor who has assessed the situation, and may be a vital precaution to safeguard someone's interests, particularly if they are involved in litigation and may be awarded compensation. (The Court of Protection is discussed further in chapter 7.)

Coping with cognitive problems

Head-injured people and their relatives frequently say they have been told that there is little that can be done to remedy the effects of brain trauma. Often it transpires that this advice was put forward by people or professionals with relatively little experience of head injury. In one respect this view is correct inasmuch as once the cells of the brain have been damaged they cannot be repaired or replaced. Immediately after head injury the neurosurgeon can stop or limit the amount of damage done to the brain by bleeding or swelling, but there is no medical treatment to repair or reconnect brain cells once they are damaged. This is not to say, however, that nothing can be done to ameliorate the effects of head injury. Structured rehabilitation provided by occupational therapists, physiotherapists, speech therapists, psychologists and doctors may well be beneficial. There is also a range of techniques and practical guidelines that can be followed, either to get around limitations or to utilise abilities that have not been damaged. In the following pages we will look at some of these techniques: some are quite straightforward, although no less useful for being so, whereas others require persistence and experimentation to get the most out of them. If you have difficulty using them, discuss the problem with a member of your rehabilitation team. Some techniques are primarily for head-injured people to use, whereas others are strategies that carers can follow. However, it is always best if both the carer and the head-injured person try these methods in a collaborative spirit and work together to overcome problems. People with cognitive problems need a good deal of encouragement, prompting and support to stick with these techniques, and by working together it is much more likely that they will be successful.

Establish a routine
One of the most helpful things that carers can do to overcome forgetfulness and confusion is to establish a regular daily rou-

tine. Most people are fairly flexible about how they fill their days, and within certain limits they get up at different times, alter mealtimes, or change their plans as necessary. In other words they adjust easily to altered circumstances or changing situations. If, however, someone has had a severe head injury and has difficulty remembering and concentrating, such variations can be confusing and irritating. A regular routine can provide a rhythm to the day and so give a sense of control, because he or she knows what to expect at any given time. If each day follows a predictable pattern the routine can cue memory, so that each event acts as a reminder of the next. Write out a daily plan of events and stick it up in a conspicuous place, such as the kitchen. Establish the habit of reviewing the diary each morning.

1 Establish a daily routine.
2 Write out a plan for each day and put it in a conspicuous place.
3 Check the plan regularly.
4 Avoid unnecessary changes in the routine.

Simplify communication

Poor or fluctuating concentration and problems with fatigue and reasoning may all mean that a head-injured person has difficulty following conversations. One of the most important things carers can do in this situation is to simplify remarks to avoid overloading or stressing the person. Speak slowly, using straightforward phrases and words, and only express one idea at a time. Check whether remarks have been understood, maybe by asking the person to repeat the information. Only then go on to talk about other topics. Likewise, when asking questions keep them simple and ask only one thing at a time: for instance, instead of asking 'Do you want chicken for today's dinner or would you prefer it tomorrow?', ask 'Do you want chicken for dinner?'. It is important to accept that communication may take time, as brain-injured people invariably process information at a slower rate than normal, besides being prone to misunderstand and make errors. Try not to get frustrated and impatient as this will only make him or her feel humiliated and will certainly not speed up matters. If someone stammers or has difficulty retrieving words, allow them time and avoid automatically providing the word. Finally, try to estimate how long he or she can concentrate on a conversation before becoming distracted or fatigued. This interval is sometimes called a person's attention span. When that time is up it is best to allow for a rest, even if it has not been possible to discuss everything. Otherwise he or she may feel you are pushing him or her too far and become irritable.

1 Simplify remarks: use simple words and phrases.
2 Express only one idea at a time.
3 Speak slowly.
4 Check that what was said has been understood by asking questions.
5 Avoid multiple questions: ask one question at a time.
6 Accept that communication may be difficult and slow: try not to be impatient or show frustration.
7 Do not exceed the person's attention span.

Use external aids and devices whenever possible

Everyone uses diaries, lists, memos, and alarms, or simply jots down notes to themselves. Aids and devices like these can also be used to overcome serious memory disorders and can be extremely useful. Perhaps the most helpful and certainly the most straightforward aid is a daily diary in which appointments, outings and tasks to be done can all be recorded. It is important to establish the habit of regularly referring to the diary throughout the day as well as jotting down problems or questions to ask later. Carers have an important role to play in this process, because a person with a severely impaired memory may forget to use the diary and need repeated reminders before it becomes routine.

There are many other similar devices such as calendars and notebooks, all of which can be useful. Check-lists can be helpful to ensure that tasks are done. This may simply consist of a sheet of paper for each day with a list of activities to be completed, written in order of priority. As each task is finished it is ticked off. The check-list should be displayed prominently, on a wall in the kitchen or bedroom, say, to make sure that it is referred to. A watch with a bleeper can be timed to go off, perhaps every half an hour, to act as a signal to check a diary or check-list, or it can be set to cue mealtimes or particular television programmes. Notes can be left in strategic places. For instance, drawers and cupboards in the kitchen can be labelled as a straightforward way of quickly identifying where things are stored. After notes have been up for a while they may be ignored, so it may be necessary to change them or use different coloured paper. There is a wide range of electronic personal organisers available commercially which can be used to store addresses and appointments and other information. Potentially these devices hold considerable promise, although they are often most useful to those with less severe cognitive problems, because people with reasoning and perceptual difficulties may find such devices too difficult to master. A dictaphone is a relatively cheap and convenient method of recording events or conversations as they arise during the day, and can be played later and the details entered into a diary.

One of the main difficulties that people with memory problems experience is getting into the habit of using these techniques consistently, and it is therefore essential for carers to play an active part in encouraging their use. Arrange a regular time, such as first thing in the morning, to review the aids and how they should be used. At first these techniques are often difficult to employ and it is easy to become disheartened if progress is not made. It is therefore important for carers to provide as much encouragement and support as possible. There are no hard and fast rules about which method to use, and it is best to experiment to see which technique or combination of techniques works for you and then stick to that.

External memory aids:
- Diaries
- Check-lists
- Notebooks
- Calendars
- Lists
- Signs and written messages
- Electronic personal organisers
- Dictaphones
- Bleep on watch

Strategies to overcome memory problems

Memory problems can sometimes be ameliorated by using mnemonic strategies, which are psychological memory aids. A mnemonic strategy is simply a way of trying to make information stick in the memory by storing it in an artificial manner. There are several strategies available and, as with external memory aids, which one to use is largely a matter of personal preference. One strategy for remembering names is to link the person's name to a visual image (face-name links). For example, to remember the name Andy Underwood, one might think of the name in terms of visual images; Andy might be remembered by thinking of a hand and a knee, and Underwood by imagining the image of a hand and a knee covered by a pile of wood. The more unusual, bizarre or amusing the image the better, since it is more likely to be retained. It can also be useful to draw the image to help it further stick in the memory. When the name has to be remembered, the person retrieves the visual image which then acts as a prompt for the name. Another technique is the Method of Loci, which is an impressive name for a straightforward strategy of linking images of objects to particular locations. For instance, to remember a shopping list of soap, deodorant and potatoes, a visual image can be formed of each of these items in a relevant location in the house. A large bar of soap can be visualised in the bathroom, a large stick of deodorant in the bedroom and a potato can be imagined filling the kitchen. When the person wants to remember each item he or she visualises each room of the house in turn and retrieves the items.

Information is invariably better retained if it is organised when we learn it. For example, it may well be difficult to remember a long shopping list if the items are written in a random order. Our recall is likely to be much better, however, if we organise the list: for instance, if the items are grouped under different headings such as dairy products, toiletries, vegetables and so on. By categorising or grouping information in this way, recall is usually much better than if no attempt is made to organise the material. Another technique suitable for young children or severely impaired adults is to include material in rhymes or short songs. An adult with severe problems and who, for example, is prone to wander off alone, can be taught a short rhyme which contains essential information such as his or her name and address. While helpful, rhymes are obviously limited as they cannot easily be adjusted to include new information. Another method to help memory retention is to rehearse the information over increasingly lengthy intervals. For instance, after telling a head-injured person someone's name, a carer can check a few seconds later whether he or she can still remember it. If so, leave it a little longer and then check again, and so on. With this technique the person has to rehearse the information over increasing lengths of time, which helps to extend gradually the duration for which information is memorised.

A technique to help written information stick in the memory is the PQRST method (PQRST stands for Preview, Question, Read, State, Test). This is a useful technique for remembering, say, a newspaper article or a piece of academic work and it consists of the following steps:

1   **Preview**: Quickly skim over the material to get a general understanding of what it is about.
2   **Question**: Ask yourself a series of questions such as what the main points of the passage are, who is the central character, what is the conclusion, and so on.
3   **Read**: Read the passage or article again, but this time bear in mind the questions you have asked yourself.
4   **State**: Repeat in your mind the material you have read and state the answers to your questions.
5   **Test**: Test your knowledge of the material at different intervals.

PQRST is useful because it provides the reader with a plan of action to follow and consequently can help reduce feelings of confusion.

Many of these techniques are different ways of getting information into the memory and helping it stay there. However, sometimes the problem is not that a person has not retained information, but that he or she has difficulty bringing it to mind: in other words, in retrieving it from memory. We all suffer from this problem occasionally, but if we receive a slight prompt everything comes back, and we can remember in detail events that for a moment had completely eluded us. In other words, we have taken the information in and retained it, but cannot momentarily get it out of the memory store. Brain damage can make retrieval particularly difficult and worsen such problems. A common technique to overcome this is to engage in mental retracing. If, for instance, you lose your car keys you will most likely form a series of visual images of where you have been since you were last in the car, and retrace your steps back to the last time you drove. By retracing what you have done, it is very often possible to identify the most likely time or place you mislaid something and thus retrieve it. People with memory problems often mislay things, and mental retracing can be a useful way of trying to identify when items were lost. Carers can also help retrieval by providing mental prompts; for instance, if a head-injured person cannot remember a name, the carer, instead of simply saying the name, can try to prompt him or her by providing the name's first letter to facilitate recall.

Mnemonic strategies, like external memory aids, all require considerable application in order to be useful, and practice and perseverance are needed if a person is to benefit. Once again, the support and encouragement of a relative or carer can be invaluable in helping someone to stick with the techniques.

Mnemonic strategies:
- Face-name links
- Method of Loci
- Organise information
- Rhymes
- Short songs
- Rehearsal
- PQRST
- Mental retracing
- First letter prompts

Learn specific tasks

It is sometimes thought that activities such as crosswords or evening classes help retrain or stimulate memory and concentration. Unfortunately there is no evidence that this is so. (This is not to say, however, that such activities are not of benefit and they may be very worthwhile for other reasons, such as to improve confidence and provide companionship.) The problem is that memory is not like a muscle which, if damaged, can be exercised and restored. When trying to overcome memory problems it is therefore better to focus on learning or relearning specific tasks, rather than trying to improve memory generally. If, for example, a person has difficulty remembering a sequence of ingredients when baking a cake, it will be more productive to try and learn that specific task (for example, by using a list), rather than rely on general mental stimulation. Having learnt how to bake a cake, one should not necessarily expect any significant improvement in remembering other recipes or other tasks. This is because people with memory problems often have difficulty in transferring what they have learnt in one area to another. One of the implications of this is that any rehabilitation or retraining should take place in or as close to the person's home as possible, because improvements made in, say, a hospital rehabilitation unit may not transfer well to other settings.

Set small and regular targets

A tendency to tire quickly is a common consequence of brain trauma. However, when people try to resume activities such as housework or hobbies, they may jump in at the deep end, and take on too much. The problem can be that they do not appreciate or anticipate the difficulties they are likely to experience and when they are not able to cope they are suddenly demoralised and lose confidence. When trying to relearn a skill it is therefore nearly always preferable to set small, achievable targets and work towards them regularly for short periods of time. As a rule, prolonged practice is unlikely to be as beneficial as working for brief intervals and then stopping for the rest of the day. By doing a little bit of work often, skills are much more likely to be acquired or relearnt. If a person is trying to relearn how to paint, for example, rather than working for several hours at a stretch it would be preferable to start by painting for maybe just half an hour every day and gradually increase this as skills and confidence return. It is important to set targets which, while relatively challenging, are nevertheless achievable, as failure only undermines confidence.

Target setting:
- Set small, achievable targets.
- Work or practise for short periods.
- Gradually increase the amount of time you are active.
- Work regularly.

Use rewards to aid learning

Overcoming cognitive problems can be frustrating for all concerned, and initially failure is more common than success. It cannot be stressed enough that rewards are essential to help you persevere with what at first can be a disheartening process. It can be helpful to set yourself small targets which, if achieved, are followed by a prearranged reward such as a trip out, a drink or a small purchase. In other words, reward yourself and acknowledge successes: this helps you focus on the fact that you are making progress and avoid negative thinking. Almost anything can be used as a reward as long as it is valued: cigarettes, special meals or snacks, are all possible rewards. Carers can play an important role in arranging rewards if someone cannot manage alone: they should generously acknowledge successes whenever they occur and provide positive feedback. The carer and the head-injured person can agree ground rules about which goals warrant a reward, and keep a record of the targets in a diary to monitor progress. If small, achievable targets have been properly agreed, the person should receive reasonably frequent rewards while working towards learning a skill: there is no point agreeing to targets that are too difficult and cannot be reached! It is just as important for carers to avoid giving negative feedback as it is to give rewards. There is a large amount of research that shows that while positive reinforcement helps people learn skills, negative feedback such as criticism, nagging or sarcasm does not spur people on and is invariably counter-productive. If someone is unable to reach a goal, or does so inconsistently, it may well be best to agree a less demanding target and pay the matter no further attention. Trying to stimulate him or her to overcome hurdles through criticism or harsh words is unlikely to be productive.

Being positive:
- Reward yourself for progress: acknowledge success.
- Carers: provide reinforcement when it is needed.
- Avoid negative feedback.

5 Emotions and personality change

In addition to cognitive problems, brain damage commonly brings about emotional, behavioural and personality changes, the precise nature and severity of which vary enormously from one person to the next. The combination of cognitive problems such as memory loss, and emotional difficulties such as lack of motivation, irritability and depression, all have a critical bearing on whether the head-injured person can get back to leading a normal life, start working again and re-establish relationships. There are a wide range of problems and in the following pages we will look at some of the more common and see how they can be overcome.

Irritability and short temper

A person who was previously reasonable and placid may become sharp-tongued and aggressive after head injury. Sensitivity to noise, a tendency to tire easily, or difficulty coping with pressure are common problems and may all precipitate outbursts of anger. A minor irritation such as a delay or a misunderstanding can cause a head-injured person to be rude or walk out. At the time it may be impossible to reason with him or her, although later, when things have cooled down, he or she may feel considerable embarrassment. Some people develop explosive tempers and are prone to severe outbursts of rage, throwing or kicking objects and even attacking people. Irritability, whether mild or severe, may be due to frustration about forgetfulness, physical limitations or financial problems, and as such may be an understandable, if unpleasant, response to such difficulties. However, it can also be the consequence of damage to the brain's mechanisms of self-control, resulting in impulsiveness and what doctors call labile emotions. Damage to the areas of the brain known as the frontal lobes is often, at least in part, responsible for such problems. The frontal lobes are located at the front of the brain behind the forehead, and it is well established that they are important for controlling emotions and for self-restraint. Because of their location they are also a common site of injury. If irritability and temper are primarily due to brain damage rather than being an emotional reaction to the person's situation, then it may be that much harder for him or her to exercise restraint and respond to demands to be reasonable. Though harder, however, it may not be impossible, and it is important not to take it for granted that such behaviour is uncontrollable, as this may only make matters worse. An important step is to identify the likely triggers for the outbursts: these may be children playing noisily, tiredness, alcohol, working too long or attempting tasks that are too demanding. Keep a note of the situations in which anger occurs in order to identify triggers and ensure that none are missed. The next step is to think of ways of dealing with the triggers. Often the best strategy is simply to avoid them: alcohol can be reduced, less demanding activities chosen or activities taken on for shorter intervals. Carers can also alter their own behaviour: misunderstandings can be reduced by simplifying communication, and carers can watch for signs of tiredness or remove noisy children. When things have calmed down, carers and the head-injured person can discuss what went wrong, identify the relevant triggers and decide how they can be avoided or minimised in future. If at all possible, carers should keep calm themselves and try not to allow themselves to be riled or feel hurt, even though such feelings may be entirely justified. It should be remembered that outbursts of temper may not be meant personally.

Anxiety and apprehension

After brain trauma there are invariably profound changes in a person's life such as unemployment, financial insecurity, uncertainty about the future and health worries. It is therefore small wonder that many people feel anxious, apprehensive and uncertain. Some develop specific fears and anxieties: if, for example, they have been in a car crash they may avoid going in cars, or when they do so they experience feelings of panic and symptoms such as palpitations and breathlessness. Fears of this intensity may well mean that the sufferer has developed a clinical phobia that requires specific psychological treatment. Cognitive problems such as forgetfulness can arouse apprehension: sufferers may worry whether they have left things unattended, or have to check that doors are locked and appliances turned off. Sometimes people become extremely obsessional and check such things repeatedly, even though they know there is no need. Physical complaints such as epilepsy can be a source of anxiety. Concerns about having a fit in public may engender considerable apprehension, as can worry about having a fit when alone.

Edward

Edward was 54 when he was run over while crossing a main road on his way to work. Afterwards he developed post-traumatic epilepsy and he also became slightly forgetful. He was a confirmed bachelor and had always lived on his own and coped satisfactorily. However, after his head injury he began to worry about having a fit at home. On two occasions he had a fit while cooking. Fortunately each time he had just turned off the gas before falling unconscious and came to no harm. After these episodes he felt panicky about the possibility of causing a fire and started to suffer from palpitations, hot sweats, and a tight feeling in his chest, all of which were symptoms of anxiety. He then began to worry about having a fit in public, and feared embarrassing himself in front of other people. Subsequently his anxieties spread and he worried about unrelated matters such as whether he could pay his bills, even though he had no real financial problems. To deal with his anxieties about cooking he bought a microwave that had an automatic timer and he replaced his stove kettle with an electric one with an automatic cut-out.

Loss and depression

Feelings of depression are extremely common as brain trauma invariably brings about many losses: loss of a job, loss of roles (such as being the breadwinner), physical limitations and cognitive limitations. Depression is only to be expected as the person becomes aware of such changes, and this is why some people, instead of getting better, feel worse as time passes after their injury. Some people experience a period of what might best be described as mourning, in much the same way as mourning occurs after a bereavement. The loss of physical and mental abilities may be keenly felt, and a period of grief for one's old life may occur before adjustment and improvement is possible.

People react in different ways, and for some depression is short-lived, whereas for others it is persistent. Usually such feelings last a matter of months before gradually subsiding. For a minority, however, depression is severe and does not lift without help. If the sufferer experiences feelings of hopelessness, believes that there is no future and starts to neglect his or her appearance, these may be signs of a significant clinical depression and relatives should be alert to the fact that medical treatment may be necessary. Loss of interest in food, difficulty getting to sleep or disturbed nights are also associated with depression. A decline in interest in sex may occur and impotence may be a problem for men. The sufferer may express ideas to the effect that life is not worth living and may talk about ending his or her life. As a rule, the more of these symptoms someone has, the more likely it is that he or she is suffering from a significant depression, and expressions of suicidal thoughts should, of course, be treated particularly seriously. In such circumstances the best course of action is for the person's GP to be asked to assess the situation. The GP may prescribe medication, as this may be the best way of bringing about improvement in the short term. A referral may also be made to a clinical psychologist or psychiatrist for a second opinion and further treatment.

Loss of interest and drive

While damage to the frontal lobes can cause aggression and impulsivity, it can also occasionally bring about the opposite effect. Instead of being excessively lively, snappy and irritable, some people seem flat and lack energy and enthusiasm. They sit around the house during the day doing little or nothing, yet nevertheless appear content with their lot and voice no complaints. Old hobbies may be neglected, or if started are soon discarded, and carers find that whenever they try to interest the person in anything, they get the reply that he or she cannot be bothered.

Frederick

After being run over while crossing a road, Frederick, a retired mechanic, changed enormously. During his retirement he had been keen on gardening and DIY, and he enjoyed decorating and doing odd jobs about the house, as well as tending his vegetable patch. Several evenings a week he went to the pub with another retired friend, and he was also a keen angler and went fishing at least once a week. After the accident, however, he became apathetic and disinterested and appeared fatigued and lacking in energy, although he never seemed particularly distressed or concerned. Although he would agree to do things for his wife they never got done, and he lost all interest in angling. He kept putting his friend off when he suggested they should go out, and in the end his friend stopped calling. He gave up gardening, and when his wife suggested he mow the lawn he replied that he would do it later, but rarely did. Occasionally he took out his tools with the intention of doing a job but the enthusiasm never lasted long and he seemed content to watch the television most of the day and stay in the house.

Apathy can be a symptom of depression and the sufferer may not do things because he or she feels too low. However, it can also occur, as in Frederick's case, without any significant lowering of mood. Some people are aware that they lack drive and specifically complain about the problem, realising that it reduces the quality of their life and prevents them studying or working. Some, however, like Frederick, have no complaints whatsoever and are content to accept a dull and repetitive routine.

Disinhibition and inappropriate behaviour

Head injury can cause disinhibition, so that the sufferer behaves in a variety of socially inappropriate or embarrassing ways with their family or in public. One of the most embarrassing is sexually inappropriate behaviour. This may be a tendency to tell suggestive jokes, laugh at vague references to sex or be over-familiar with members of the opposite sex. One young man, for example, had a tendency to stand a little too close to women and he frequently touched their arms or put his hand on their shoulders while talking. Although his behaviour did not cause serious offence, there was no doubt that most women found it off-putting. Another man was far less constrained and he took to writing long, sexually explicit scripts which he then sent to members of his family and to publishers. He frequently referred to sexual matters in conversation and was indifferent to people's embarrassment. In fact he seemed to enjoy their consternation and no amount of reasoning from his parents could persuade him to stop.

A preoccupation with sex is unsurprising, as many head-injured people are teenagers or young adults for whom sex is, in any event, a major interest. While sexual disinhibition is perhaps the most striking form of inappropriate behaviour, disinhibition is not restricted to sexual matters and there are a wide range of potential problems. It can take the form of talking too loudly; commenting rudely on other people; wearing odd combinations of clothes; or laughing on a sad occasion. Childishness and demanding behaviour can be particularly embarrassing, and many partners find such behaviour especially difficult to tolerate. Disinhibition is often associated with a loss of insight, so that the head-injured person has no real appreciation that his or her behaviour is inappropriate and so makes no effort to change. Moreover, they may be quite unable to learn that their conduct is unacceptable, despite being told so by their relatives, and occasionally such feedback perversely exacerbates the problem.

Coping with emotional problems

As with cognitive problems, head-injured people and their relatives are often told that there is little that can be done to overcome emotional and personality changes after brain trauma. However, as with cognitive problems, this is incorrect and such advice is simply the counsel of despair! As we know, the brain itself cannot be repaired but this does not mean that it is impossible to learn new skills or that limitations cannot be circumvented. Problems such as irritability and depression are, in any event, rarely exclusively - or even always partly - due to brain damage. Rather they may result from many other factors such as loss of friends, inactivity and loneliness, physical restrictions and so on. In order to cope with these problems the head-injured person may turn to alcohol or drugs, which create further complications such as arguments at home, marital strife or financial problems. There is nearly always something which can be done to minimise or overcome these problems, and new ways of dealing with stress and emotional difficulties can be learnt. In the following pages we will look at a number of straightforward but nevertheless effective strategies which can be used to lessen these problems.

Keeping active

An extremely important and simple way of coping with feelings of anxiety and depression is to keep active. Many people slip into a state of inactivity after head injury, sometimes because during recuperation they do relatively little and later do not get back to an active routine; and sometimes because they are encouraged to take it easy by relatives and friends. More commonly it is because they lack drive and initiative and feel too low or apathetic to be bothered with socialising and going out, and think they will get back to doing things when they feel better. However, inactivity nearly always makes emotional problems worse, and rather than waiting until feelings of depression lift before doing more, it is important to do more to make the depression lift.

Even in the worst of cases, it is unlikely that there is nothing a person can do after head injury. The important thing is to identify enjoyable and satisfying activities to engage in on a regular basis. Decorating a room is fine, but once done it cannot be done again, and it is therefore preferable to identify activities that can be done regularly, such as attending a weekly group. Local colleges offer recreational and academic courses which may be suitable, and voluntary organisations and charities are nearly always grateful for any help, even if it is only a few hours a week. Libraries, health centres, local authorities and Citizens' Advice Bureaux can provide information on local amenities. In Britain the National Head Injuries Association (Headway) has local groups in most parts of the country which meet regularly and organise social events and talks by professionals and carers about head injury. Such groups are an invaluable source of support (the address of the national organising body is provided at the end of this book). Of course, not all activities have to be outside the home, and resuming old hobbies such as reading or sewing can be an important step. After identifying a number of different activities, draw up a plan for each day of the week and write down when and for how long each activity is to be done, ticking each one off when it is completed. This helps overcome forgetfulness and ensures that you do each activity. It makes sense to set a modest pace at first, with perhaps an upper limit of a few hours' activity a day initially. After a week or two, as the activities become routine, more can be added and a range of different pursuits progressively built into the plan. By pacing the number of activities and taking things slowly but steadily, it is likely that better progress will be made than if a lot of activities are taken on all at once. Perseverance is likely to be repaid with improved confidence and an improvement in mood.

Becoming active:
1 Write out a list of enjoyable, regular activities to do inside and outside the home.
2 Draw up a daily programme specifying when and for how long each activity is to be done.
3 Check the programme regularly to ensure each day's activities are completed. Tick each one when it is done.
4 Gradually increase the number of activities.

Problem-solving and dealing with negative thinking

A large body of research has shown that distressing feelings such as anxiety and depression often stem from negative ways of thinking. For example, feeling low may result from the belief that the future is hopeless, that the head injury is a punishment or that facial scars are noticeable to everyone. Such thoughts, if they go unchallenged, can cause depression because they are essentially negative ways of thinking about life and the future. When someone feels depressed or hopeless it usually also becomes harder for them to think more positive thoughts to counteract their negative ideas, and at the same time it becomes steadily easier to think other pessimistic and self-destructive thoughts. In other words, thinking becomes subtly distorted and the combination of increasingly negative thoughts and difficulty in remembering positive ideas sets up a downward spiral that ends in a profound feeling of worry or depression. A person who thinks that scars on his or her face are very noticeable and

unsightly may, for example, avoid socialising to prevent embarrassment. However, loss of companionship may lead to despondency and an erosion of confidence so that they become
more conscious of their appearance, and avoid socialising all the
more. In other words, avoidance makes things worse. In this
situation it would be better to take the opposite approach and
make a particular effort to socialise, while deliberately thinking
positive, confidence-building thoughts (for example 'No one
really pays that much attention to my scars', 'The scars are
hardly noticeable'). By deliberately bringing to mind positive
ideas or counter-arguments it may be possible to obtain a more
balanced perspective of the situation.

A useful technique is to record negative thoughts as they
occur in a diary or notebook. Often one negative thought leads
to another, so that upsetting thoughts about, say, having epilepsy lead on to further pessimistic thoughts about being unemployed or not having friends. It is important to write down every
one, so that all the upsetting ideas are clearly set out. Having
identified the distressing thoughts, the next step is to write
down positive counter-arguments. At this stage ask yourself a
number of questions:

1 What is the evidence in support of this belief or idea?
2 What other way is there of looking at the situation?
3 Even if the negative thought is true, what can I do to
   overcome the problem?

By thinking coolly and dispassionately about the problem it
may be possible to recognise that things are not as they first
appear to be, and there are other ways of looking at the situation. For instance, the idea 'I'm useless to my partner now I'm
not working' could be answered by checking whether it is true
that you are really 'useless' or whether, despite being unemployed, there are other things you do to help apart from work.
Activities such as washing-up, tidying the house, laying the
table and shopping may all be worthwhile and, although not the
same as going to work, may nevertheless be important and
appreciated. These activities should be written down to put the
negative idea in perspective. The next step is to ask the second
question: is there another way of looking at the situation? In
this case a new and more constructive response might be to say
something like 'Sure I'm not working, but I'm doing as much as
I can to help'. It may be helpful to write this down as well, so

that this new way of thinking is not forgotten and can be referred to later. It is important to recognise that thinking positively does not mean that one should deny that problems exist. Indeed, the opposite is true. As in this example, problems should be acknowledged, because trying to pretend that they are not there is unlikely to be convincing. Nor does positive thinking mean saying something vaguely encouraging to yourself such as 'Everything will work out all right'. Rather, it involves developing a sense of perspective so that the good, as well as the bad, aspects of a situation are recognised.

Sometimes a situation is undeniably bad, and far from being overly pessimistic a very real problem has been accurately recognised. In this case the problem should again be written down in full and then tackled by asking the third question listed above: what can be done about it? Let us take another example to illustrate this approach. The thought 'I've lost all my friends since my head injury' may be true, as many people find that their social life dwindles after brain trauma. If so, it is only to be expected that someone in this situation will feel despondent. However, because a depressing thought is correct does not mean that it has to be accepted as unchangeable. On the contrary, the next step is to think of practical solutions to change the situation. In this case one way forward would be to decide to get into situations where you are likely to meet other people and develop a social life. Depending on your preferences and what is available this could involve joining a social club, going to college or joining a self-help group. Let us say that your preference is to join a group. To do this might require some intermediate steps such as finding out from a local library which groups meet in your area. If you have problems with mobility then another step would be to arrange transport. By working through the problem in this practical way a plan of action can be developed and then followed through to solve the problem. It can be helpful to write down each step, which in this case might consist of the following:

- **Step one**: Go to the library tomorrow and ask about local social and self-help groups.
- **Step two**: Draw up a list of groups that sound interesting and phone and ask for further information.
- **Step three**: Discuss with the social worker whether transport could be arranged.

Here the first step towards overcoming the loss of friends is to go to the library the next day. Clearly this is just a first step, and much more will be required before the original negative thought is finally addressed. Nevertheless, even deciding to take that first step makes many people feel much more positive and in charge of their lives, and with each further step their confidence grows. Drawing up a practical plan of action has the advantage that you know when you are working to solve a problem and so making progress, and when you are not, and this can be a useful spur to action.

Below are some further examples of negative thoughts which many head-injured people have from time to time. Often people accept such ideas as being obviously correct or unalterable, and consequently consider the fact that they are depressed or anxious as inevitable and unchangeable. As we shall see, however, many negative thoughts are not really as true or as accurate as they initially appear to be, and even when a situation is correctly appraised that does not mean it cannot be changed.

Negative thought: 'Everyone thinks I'm mad because I've got epilepsy.'
Positive challenges: A negative thought like this can be challenged by asking yourself, is it true? In reply you could say: 'No, not everyone thinks this, in fact, no one I know has said I'm crazy. It's because I feel anxious and self-conscious that I'm feeling this way'. Is there another way of looking at the situation? 'Yes, only a few people think epilepsy is a sign of madness and they only think that because they don't understand it. Most people aren't even aware I suffer from epilepsy at all.' What can be done about the situation? 'Relax, I'm worrying unnecessarily. I'll try to think about my condition less, then I won't be so self-conscious about it.'

Negative thought: 'I'm so forgetful it's embarrassing, people think I'm stupid.'
Positive challenges: Is it true? 'It's true I'm forgetful and that I get embarrassed about it, but do people think I'm stupid? No, most people react very well when I forget things and no one has been impatient or laughed. I'm just assuming they think that way when there is no evidence that they do.' Is there another way of looking at the situation? 'Yes, I feel embarrassed because

I think people think I'm stupid, but there's no need to feel like that.' What can be done about the situation? 'My real problem is not other people, it's my forgetfulness. I'll make more effort to use my diary and memory techniques to get around the problem.'

Negative thought: 'I'll never work again, I've got no future.'
Positive challenges: Is this true? 'It's true that I won't be able to go back to my old job because of my muscle weakness, but does that mean I've got no future at all? No, there are many other things that I can do apart from work.' Is there another way of looking at the situation? 'I may not be able to work but I've got many other things going for me. I need to think differently about the future and make new plans.' What can be done about the situation? 'I'll make sure I have got a future. I've always fancied taking some courses at college and I'll make some enquiries. I could also see if there are any voluntary groups locally that need help and see what I can offer.'

Negative thought: 'Nobody will look at me now, I'll never go out with anyone in this state.'
Positive challenges: Is it true? 'It's true I'm not going out with anyone at the moment, but that doesn't mean I never will. Plenty of people with head injuries and disabilities go out with people, why should I be any different?' Is there another way of looking at the situation? 'If I can get on with my family and friends, why shouldn't I get on with someone of the opposite sex once they get to know me?' What can be done about the situation? 'I need to go out more and get in touch with people and then I might meet someone. I'll ring up some of my old friends and arrange to see them, and I'll see if there are any drop-in centres I can go to.'

Negative thought: 'I lost everything when I had that accident.'
Positive challenges: Is this true? 'Did I really lose everything? No, I lost my job, but I didn't lose other things that are much more important to me, like my children and family.' Is there another way of looking at the situation? 'My life has certainly changed in some areas since the accident, but many things are the same. I mustn't think everything has changed when it hasn't, because that will only get me down.' What can be

done about the situation? 'I'll write out a list of things that haven't changed and that I cope with normally, so that I get things into perspective.'

Negative thought: 'I can't concentrate properly to study, I'm useless.'
Positive challenges: Is this true? 'I definitely can't concentrate on my work as well as I did, that's true.' Is there another way of looking at the situation? 'I'm going to have to come to terms with the fact that my concentration is poor, but that doesn't mean I'm useless and, in fact, I'm coping well with many other aspects of my life'. What can be done about the situation? 'I should stop calling myself useless, it only makes me depressed and it's not true. I'll think about changing courses to something a bit more practical to get around the problem.'

By writing out negative thoughts and then challenging them in this way, it may be possible either to reject them as incorrect, or see that while they have some correct aspects, they nevertheless exaggerate the situation. Alternatively, they may be true and it may be understandable to feel worried or depressed. However, even if a situation is upsetting it is rarely ever completely unchangeable, and the next step is therefore to work towards change.

Learning to relax
Feelings of anxiety and tension are common after head injury and, apart from being unpleasant in their own right, may bring on or worsen other complaints. Headaches, muscular aches and pains, disturbed sleep, poor appetite and epileptic fits are just some of the many complaints that can stem from, or be worsened by, stress and anxiety. Learning to control anxiety is therefore an important way of controlling symptoms and developing a sense of well-being. Some people turn to alcohol to help them relax because alcohol relaxes the nervous system and so reduces unpleasant physical symptoms such as tremulousness, rapid heart beat and sweating. The hazards of drinking are well known and it is clearly not a constructive way of tackling stress since it does not alter underlying problems. For the head-injured person alcohol poses particular risks, since after a brain injury a person's tolerance is often diminished, and even small

quantities of drink can cause intoxication and hence worsen other problems such as disinhibited behaviour. Long-term excessive drinking will also further damage the brain and worsen cognitive problems such as memory loss and diminished concentration.

There are many self-help techniques that can be used to control anxiety and stress, and two particularly effective techniques, **Progressive Relaxation** and **Controlled Breathing**, will be described in the pages that follow. Progressive Relaxation is a simple, straightforward method of controlling tension and because no drugs are involved there are no side-effects and, of course, no danger of addiction. Most importantly it puts the person using it in control, since it is what he or she does that brings about the improvement. At first the feeling of relaxation may only last a short while, but providing the exercise is practised regularly, the ability to relax becomes more profound and lasts longer.

To be effective Progressive Relaxation requires commitment, as improvement is not instantaneous but rather a gradual process. Most people practise Progressive Relaxation for several weeks and months, and as they do so they learn to deepen their relaxation response, as well as use it to tackle stresses that crop up in their daily routine. The exercise takes about twenty to twenty-five minutes and should be completed at least once a day. As a rule it is far more likely to be effective if it is practised regularly on a daily basis than if it is practised several times one day and then not at all for a few days. Before starting Progressive Relaxation take the following steps:

1 Choose a quiet room such as a bedroom where you can be sure not to be disturbed for about twenty to twenty-five minutes.
2 Sit in a comfortable chair that has a head-rest or lie on a bed or on the floor with a pillow under your head. Sit or lie so that all parts of your body are supported by the chair, bed or floor.
3 Close your eyes and collect your thoughts and take a few moments to sit or lie still. Do not rush.

Progressive Relaxation consists of the following three stages. Take them in turn and do not hurry. If you have finished the exercise in less than twenty minutes, that is too fast and next time you must slow down. At first time the session until it becomes routine.

Progressive Relaxation

Stage one
This stage consists of breathing naturally and taking a few moments to rest. Do nothing and clear your mind in preparation for Progressive Relaxation.

1   Attend to your breathing. Breathe in and out naturally. Just let it happen for a minute or two.

Stage two
This stage consists of tensing and relaxing various parts of your body. When tensing muscles, do not bring on any pain or discomfort. It is important to breathe in when tensing muscles and breathe out when relaxing. When you relax, exhale all at once and let all the tension go. Say 'relax' in your mind when you exhale, so that unwinding is associated with saying 'relax' to yourself. Afterwards reflect on the feelings of relaxation and appreciate how the muscles feel heavy and warm.

2   Start first with your **hands**. Clench both hands to form a fist and at the same time breathe in. Hold the tension for about five seconds, breathing naturally. Concentrate on the tension. Then relax the hands and breathe out. Say 'relax' to yourself. Let your hands go limp and loose. After a few moments tense your hands again and repeat the exercise.

3   Next turn your attention to your **forearms**, the lower arms. Tense your forearms by bending your hands at your wrists so that your hands point up. Breathe in. Hold the tension for five seconds, breathing normally. Then let go, breathe out, and say 'relax'. Notice the difference between tension and relaxation. Breathe normally. Rest a few moments and then tense your forearms again.

4   Focus on your biceps muscles, the **upper arms**. Tense these muscles by breathing in and touching your shoulders with your fists. Hold the tension for five seconds, breathing normally. Then breathe out and say 'relax'. Breathe normally again. Notice that the muscles begin to feel warm and heavy. After a few moments' rest repeat the exercise.

5 The next set of muscles are the **shoulders**. This time lift your shoulders to your ears. Hold it for five seconds, and then relax. Rest a few moments and then repeat the action.

6 Now concentrate on your facial muscles. This time raise your **eyebrows** as if you were surprised. Hold it for five seconds, and when you let go, exhale and say 'relax'. Rest a few moments and then repeat the step.

7 The next step involves tensing several face muscles at the same time. Wrinkle your **nose** tightly, press your **lips** together and press your **tongue** into the roof of your mouth. Hold it for five seconds. Breathe out and let go, saying 'relax'. After a rest, repeat the procedure.

8 Next breathe in so that your **chest** expands like a barrel. Hold it for five seconds and then let out the breath and let the tension go. Breathe normally again for a few moments and then breathe in again. Hold it for five seconds and then let go of the tension.

9 Focus now on your **stomach**. Brace your stomach muscles as if you were expecting a punch. Hold the tension again for five seconds, then let it go all at once. Repeat the step.

10 This time lift your legs slightly off the ground, bed or floor to tense your **thighs**. Repeat after a brief rest.

11 The last step is to tense your **lower legs** by curling your toes up into the air and pressing your feet down into the floor or bed. Repeat and remember to let all the tension go.

Stage three
When you have completed Progressive Relaxation do not get up immediately, but take a few moments to reflect on the session.

12 Check through your body to see if there are still any feelings of tension. If so, repeat the exercise for that part of the body.

13 Continue to breathe naturally. When you breathe out, say 'relax'.

14 Focus on the difference between tension and relaxation. Become familiar with recognising even low levels of tension.

An important part of learning to relax is recognising when there is a build-up of tension in response to problems and stresses that arise during the day. A slight increase in tension can be used as a signal to practise Progressive Relaxation and so stop a build-up in anxiety before it reaches a point where it is difficult to control. Some people find particular parts of Progressive Relaxation more helpful than others, and just practising those may be sufficient, whereas on another occasion it may be necessary to complete the whole exercise. A build-up in tension can also be used to prompt you to start identifying any worrying, negative thoughts that are causing the tension, and then challenge them in the way outlined earlier.

Controlled Breathing exercises

Anxiety and worried feelings can cause hyperventilation. The term 'hyperventilation' means overbreathing or, to put it more straightforwardly, breathing too quickly.

Hyperventilation can easily be detected because the chest rises and falls and often there is a feeling of being out of breath. Although the problem may be obvious to others, however, many people who hyperventilate are not themselves aware of what they are doing. This may be because irregular breathing has become a habit and, like any other habit, tends to occur automatically. How then can you tell if you are breathing wrongly? There are a number of signs to look for. Pay attention to your breathing and check whether it is rapid and irregular, particularly in response to stress. Physical symptoms such as dizziness and faintness, and sensations like pins and needles in your hands or legs may also indicate that you are hyperventilating. Another sign is whether the top of your chest rises and falls during breathing instead of your stomach moving in and out. If your stomach moves in and out, then you are breathing properly, using the part of your body called the diaphragm. If, however, your chest rises and falls, you are breathing incorrectly and not properly emptying and filling your lungs.

Overcoming hyperventilation involves relearning how to breathe in a controlled, regular pattern. As with Progressive Relaxation the technique is quite straightforward, although it requires practice. Set aside a regular time to go through the exercise and complete it in a quiet room where you will not be disturbed. Ensure that you are warm and comfortable. Lie on a bed or on the floor, or sit in a chair.

- **Step one. Diaphragmatic breathing**: breathe from the abdomen, so that when you breathe your stomach moves in and out, instead of your chest rising and falling.
- **Step two. Breathe evenly**: make sure that each breath in is as long as each breath out. Avoid short, rapid, irregular breaths. Count slowly to yourself when you breathe in and out, and try to reach the same number each time.
- **Step three. Breathe slowly**: gradually slow down the time it takes to breathe in and out, so that you take fewer breaths per minute. This takes practice and should not be rushed.

Practising how to breathe may seem strange at first because breathing, of course, is something that we take for granted. It can also be quite difficult, and initially some people find that instead of getting better, their breathing gets worse. This is because paying attention to breathing can be disruptive until one gets used to it. Another reason is that some people try too hard to slow their breathing and force the pace of progress, so making themselves breathless. With practice these problems fade and gradually an even breathing rhythm establishes itself.

Medication for emotional problems

Sometimes feelings of depression and hopelessness are so over-whelming that it seems too difficult to try to do more or stop negative thinking. Strong feelings of anxiety with unpleasant symptoms such as palpitations can also occasionally be difficult to control. In these circumstances your doctor may recommend that you take an antidepressant or tranquilliser. Nowadays, and with good reason, many people are wary of taking tablets as a way of solving emotional problems as they are afraid of becoming dependent and suffering side-effects and they appreciate that ultimately medicines will not alter underlying problems. Nevertheless it is important not to dismiss such treatment too quickly, as it can have an important role to play in overcoming distressing feelings. An antidepressant, for example, may be a useful way of lightening mood and so providing the motivation to start taking on new activities that otherwise seem too much. Once some progress has been made and confidence begins to increase, the antidepressant can be gradually withdrawn. In this way, medication taken for a limited period can play an invaluable role. The main concern that many people have about antidepressants and tranquillisers is that they might end up taking them indefinitely. Whilst this occurred in the past, doctors are increasingly aware of the need to review whether patients need their medication, and so the likelihood of remaining on a course of treatment indefinitely has greatly diminished. Which medicine to take and for how long are questions you should discuss with your doctor, so that you can come to a joint decision about the type of treatment that is right for you.

6 Head injury is a family affair

The American psychologist Muriel Lezak has said that head injury is a family affair: that is, the effects of head injury are not limited to the brain trauma victim but other people – partner, children or parents – may all be affected and need to adjust to having a disabled relative and cope with the resulting problems. As the majority of head-injured people are men, if they are in a relationship it is their partner who usually has to shoulder these problems. If the person is single they may be discharged to their parents once hospital care is completed, and the latter will have to adjust to having a dependent son or daughter again.

In the immediate aftermath of the accident when the victim is still in hospital, relatives are only concerned with whether he or she will survive. This is understandable: they may be in a state of shock and anxiety and the only thing that matters is that their loved one pulls through. When it becomes clear the patient will survive, attention shifts to other matters such as getting him or her mobile, toileting, feeding and so on. Relatives have an important role to play in helping the rehabilitation team, and in the early weeks and months there can be impressive improvements that may promise a good outcome. Relief coupled with a desire to help the nurses and staff may take up all their attention and energy. As well as these immediate concerns there are often a host of other issues to deal with, such as running a home, working, and looking after children. Eventually, however, things start to settle down and about six months to a year after the head injury, many relatives begin to take stock of the situation. The anniversary of the head injury can be an important time for reflection, as it is about then that it begins to be possible to judge what the long-term situation is likely to be.

What do relatives find stressful?

What are the main problems that relatives experience? Most people who do not personally care for a head-injured person can easily understand that being a carer is likely to be stressful, and identify problems such as lifting and carrying, incontinence and feeding difficulties as the most likely sources of stress. However, most research studies show that this is not the case and while relatives do not relish such tasks, they are quite prepared to deal with them. By and large the most stressful difficulties are the psychological changes in the sufferer; that is, cognitive problems such as forgetfulness and loss of concentration, and personality changes entailing childishness and embarrassing behaviour. The following are some of the most common problems from the perspective of a group of relatives who took part in a research study in Scotland:

• Irritability
• Impatience
• Tiredness
• Poor memory

The most frequently reported symptoms were the cognitive and emotional disturbances, and complaints about physical disability were far less common. These psychological problems tend to be seen by carers as more distressing because their loved one is no longer the same, and they have to adjust to living with a sometimes very different person. One research study conducted in Israel illustrated the problems that relatives experience by comparing the responses of wives of brain trauma patients with the wives of men who had suffered damage to the spinal cord, but who had no head injury. Both groups of men had suffered serious injuries which had profoundly changed their lives, and their partners had to adjust to major changes in their relationships. However, the partners of the head-injured were nevertheless more depressed, and described their lives as having changed more than the partners in the other group. They also felt lonely and isolated and had taken on their husbands' roles. Clearly, looking after a head-injured person is uniquely stressful.

It is sometimes thought that particular family members experience a greater sense of burden from looking after a head-injured person than others. Women looking after a head-injured partner have been thought to suffer more stress than parents looking after a head-injured son. This is because it is assumed that parents have less difficulty resuming a caring role, whereas a woman who has had no expectation of having to nurse her partner and run the household single-handed may find the strain too much. While this view has an intuitive appeal, in practice it is unproductive trying to estimate who suffers most. In any event there are many exceptions to these generalisations and some women cope admirably and adjust well to the new situation, whereas some parents who may have been looking forward to having more time to themselves do not. Parents may cope well initially but become less able to manage as time passes and they themselves become infirm. Elderly parents, in particular, often worry about the future and how their invalid relative will cope when they are no longer alive.

Acknowledging feelings

Living with a severely head-injured person can arouse many different emotions, some of which may be difficult to come to terms with, although all are understandable.

- **Disgust**: when dealing with toileting or incontinence, or during sex.
- **Fear**: of the head-injured person's temper, or concerning safety about the house, or in response to fits.
- **Annoyance**: about forgetfulness and repetitive questions.
- **Embarrassment**: about silly remarks or inappropriate behaviour in public or in front of friends.
- **Anger**: at ingratitude for care provided.
- **Envy**: of friends or relatives who do not have to look after someone who has been injured.
- **Depression and worry**: because of loneliness and anxiety about the future.
- **Loss and grief**: for the partner or child who has now changed.
- **Guilt**: for having these feelings, or for wanting to be alone.

It may be difficult to accept such emotions let alone admit them to others, although they are in fact quite common. It is important for carers not to feel that they are abnormal or selfish for having such feelings, or that others in a similar situation necessarily feel differently. The truth is that many carers have mixed feelings about caring. Talking to other carers or relatives can be extremely valuable in helping to come to terms with these emotions, as it will show that most have experienced similar responses at some time. Sometimes carers feel quite angry and hostile because of the demands placed upon them, and when pushed to the limit they want to hit or punish the person, or handle him or her aggressively. Again, many people react this way and such feelings are not uncommon. What this means is that the carer has come to the end of their ability to cope and needs help. It is important to discuss these problems with a GP or social worker and work out a solution together. It may be that a period of respite care is needed or more regular help in the home. Alternatively the best solution might be for the head-injured person to live in a place where there are professional helpers who are better placed to cope with the demands of caring. The important thing is not to struggle on alone but to acknowledge these problems and then discuss what can be done to overcome them.

Changing roles and relationships

Having a head-injured partner or child at home nearly always brings about changes in the carer's life, and not uncommonly these changes are profound. The carer may no longer be able to go to work because he or she has to look after the head-injured victim. Alternatively a woman who has never been employed may be forced to go out to work because her partner is unemployed. A carer may have to take on several roles and act as nurse, wage-earner and child-raiser, besides dealing with all the routine chores involved in running the house such as paying the bills, cooking and washing and coping with emergencies. A common problem is loneliness as it may not be possible to confide in one's partner and share difficulties, and so many problems have to be faced alone. Anybody who has had to give up work is deprived at a stroke of important social contacts, as well as other rewards that come from a career. If the head-injured person has suffered a change in personality, friends and relatives who were initially supportive and visited regularly may begin to call less frequently, and many carers say that friends just dwindle away. This is perhaps understandable, if not inevitable, if the person is aggressive or disinhibited, but it obviously leaves the carer isolated and forced to cope alone. Tied to caring for someone who is handicapped, or physically well but psychologically changed, it may be difficult, if not impossible, to go out and have a life outside the home, particularly if there are young children to look after.

The financial costs of looking after someone with a head injury can be daunting, particularly in the United States where medical care is provided largely by the private sector. One American study concluded that when the costs of medical bills, medication, rehabilitation, legal fees and numerous other expenses are calculated, together with loss of income through unemployment, the total amount is staggering. In Britain, where acute medical care is free and therefore not a financial concern, there may nevertheless be many other expenses such as the cost of special aids, modifications to the house and other requirements. Specialised rehabilitation for psychological problems is largely unavailable within the National Health Service and may only be obtained in the private sector at considerable cost, with most private units charging well beyond the means of most people. As such rehabilitation usually continues for many months, the total bill may be colossal, and consequently unaffordable by most families. Some of these expenses may be met as part of a compensation claim, but for those not eligible to make a claim it may be impossible to recoup such costs.

Even in these more enlightened times many couples still organise their relationships along relatively traditional lines and while both partners may go to work the man still takes the more dominant role in making financial and family decisions while the woman largely retains responsibility for the home. After head injury this may change and there can be a significant reversal of roles. Intellectual impairment may mean that the man is unable to work or do odd jobs about the house, with the result that his partner has to take on tasks she never anticipated. This role reversal may be difficult for both partners: the head-injured man may feel that he has lost face because he is dependent and has to be looked after, whereas the woman has to cope with the strain of making family decisions alone that previously she expected to share. Instead of having an ally, women sometimes say that it is like having another child to look after, and they feel they have become caretakers instead of equal partners. Embarrassing behaviour in a previously mature man, as well as dependency and temper outbursts all inevitably have an impact on a relationship and may erode past affection.

Sexual problems

Sexual problems are by no means uncommon after head injury. Many victims of brain trauma lose interest in sex and suffer what doctors call a loss of libido (a reduced sex drive). Alternatively the opposite problem may present itself: the person is easily aroused and preoccupied with sex, frequently demanding intercourse and insensitive to their partner's wishes (this is called hypersexuality). They may be crude and disinhibited, and make inappropriate remarks no matter how embarrassing. The causes of these problems vary, although both excessive interest or loss of interest can result from damage to the frontal lobes of the brain. Physical limitations such as muscular weakness which make it difficult to adopt the positions for sex can affect a person's sex drive. Loss of interest can also be a symptom of emotional problems such as anxiety and depression. Anxiety in women can cause dryness in the vagina and consequently pain during intercourse. In men it can cause impotence (inability to achieve or sustain an erection). Impotence may cause the sufferer to become anxious about how he will perform the next time he has sex, so that this apprehension itself causes further impotence. He may then find himself in a vicious circle where impotence causes anxiety, which in turn causes further impotence.

These problems inevitably affect the uninjured partner who finds that sex becomes a chore he or she dislikes and avoids. This may be because the warmth and intimacy previously shared with their partner is no longer there, and they feel that he or she is no longer the same person. It can also be difficult, if not impossible, for a couple to switch from having a dependant-carer relationship to having an equal and adult sexual relationship, with the effect that their sex life dwindles. As we have seen, being a carer can be extremely stressful and if the carer feels tense or depressed, his or her own emotional state can affect their sex drive. If this is the case their interest may only pick up if or when the underlying stresses are relieved.

Impact on the children

It is not only adults who have to adjust to having a head-injured relative; often there are children who have to adjust as well. A toddler may not take in what has happened and be relatively unaffected, but a child at primary school can be very aware that their parent has changed and be frightened by tempers and unpredictability. Behavioural problems may be copied, mocked or viewed as a source of embarrassment, or alternatively the child may come to treat their parent like a child. Such reactions are understandable, although inevitably they create further problems for the other parent who has to divide his or her attention between a partner and the children. Older children may want to shoulder some of the burden and become involved in the day-to-day running of the house and help look after their head-injured parent. This can be a positive development, as the child can benefit by becoming more mature and understanding. However, a balance must be struck so that children are not drawn so far into a caring role that their own development through their social lives and education is affected.

The following steps can help to minimise the impact of a parent's head injury:

1 Explain what is wrong: children need to understand why their father or mother is short-tempered or irritable, or why he or she cannot remember things properly. If they do not know that their father shouts and swears because he has suffered brain damage, the whole situation may be frightening and feel out of control. In this respect children are just like adults, and if they have the situation explained to them they are far less likely to be fearful of it. Informing and educating children that their father is short-tempered, not because they have done something wrong or because he dislikes them, but because he is ill, will help reduce their anxiety. Remember it is surprising how much even a young child can understand if it is explained in a simple and straightforward manner.

2 Carers can schedule time for children and their injured

parent to spend together. This may just be a case of them going shopping regularly or watching a football match, and need not necessarily consist of particularly special or unusual activities. It is important to arrange activities that are sure to be successful. If, for instance, the injured person suffers from irritability, ensure that he or she is not put in a position that may provoke them, such as a noisy environment. If the activity passes off successfully, this is likely to be good for both the parent and the children, and the more everyday activities are maintained, the stronger the relationship between children and parent is likely to be.

3 Make a particular point of checking that the children carry on with their usual activities. If they are going out regularly to scouts, or ballet classes, or visiting their friends, they are doing what other children usually do and leading normal lives. If they stop any of these activities it may be necessary to make a particular point of encouraging them to resume them.

4 Check how they are getting on at school. If, for any reason, a child is having problems at home this often shows itself first by a drop in performance at school. Discuss their school progress and behaviour with their teachers in order to identify any problems at an early stage. If there are problems these can then be talked about at home and worries about either parent can be addressed.

Separation and divorce

Some couples survive head injury well, and indeed some come to feel that the trauma they have undergone has brought them closer together. Unfortunately, however, it has to be said that such couples are not in the majority and most experience some strain, and for many that strain becomes intolerable. Studies of marriages where one partner has had a brain injury suggest that marital distress is commonplace and the incidence of divorce is higher than normal. The dilemma for a wife or husband caught in a marriage that has irreparably changed can be profound. The psychologist Muriel Lezak has pointed out that not only must the uninjured spouse face up to the fact that their partner has altered and hence they may not wish to continue the relationship, but he or she also has to square it with their conscience to leave their invalid partner. Unfortunately there may be no socially acceptable way to do this and, caught between their conscience, past affection and the present situation a husband or wife may feel trapped in a loveless marriage from which there seems to be no escape.

There is, of course, no easy way out of this dilemma. Perhaps the first step is to acknowledge that the problem exists, as it may be difficult even to admit this for fear of seeming to be disloyal. Having admitted that there is a problem the next step is often to discuss it with someone else, possibly members of the family or friends, although as they are probably involved in the situation themselves, they may not be able to listen dispassionately and give objective advice. An outside professional, such as a family doctor or social worker, may be preferable. A counsellor can help explore the options, although it should be borne in mind that while counsellors are skilled in advising on relationships, they may have relatively little experience of the unique problems that follow head injury. Discussion may help clarify feelings and issues, and allow the development of a plan for the future which takes everyone's interests into account. It may be that separation and divorce are the result. While distressing, if the separation takes place in an organised manner, then arrangements can be made with the professionals involved to minimise the pain for everyone.

Reducing the stress of caring

As we have seen, having a head-injured partner or relative can be physically and mentally stressful and place considerable burdens upon the carer and wider family. To cope with what may be a long-term commitment it is therefore essential for carers to have the opportunity to meet their own needs for rest and relaxation, and continue to have a life apart from caring. In the pages that follow we will outline some straightforward guidelines to help minimise the strain. These guidelines are not original and most people acknowledge that they are likely to be helpful. However, the problem for many carers is not that they do not know how to reduce stress, but rather that they ignore their own needs, feeling that the other person's requirements take precedence. Unfortunately in the long run this is likely to result in a build-up in stress until the burden of caring becomes intolerable. Use these guidelines as a check-list to see where changes can be made to minimise the strain.

Setting limits

Survivors of head injury can be extremely demanding and expect everything to be done for them, sometimes because they need reassurance, or because brain damage causes their behaviour to regress. Traumatised themselves by what has happened, relatives can be overprotective and worry about fits and falls and prefer to take on tasks such as lifting or preparing meals. Gradually they can find themselves doing more and more, and the net effect is that they become overwhelmed and unable to cope. It is therefore important to set limits and there are two kinds of limit to set: first, limits for the carer; and second, limits for the head-injured person.

To limit the amount of work done it can be helpful to draw up a list of jobs that have to be done and those which it would be nice to do, but which are not essential. For example, it may be necessary to accompany the injured person to the doctor, or ensure that medication is taken on time, but there may be other tasks which are not as important, such as tidying the house every day, or cooking every meal. Review which tasks are essential and which are optional or can even be left out. Having identified what has to be done, it is also important to work through these tasks at a reasonable rate; in other words, it is important for carers to pace themselves. Many people think that, as a good carer, they have to do everything at once, or that if they have time on their hands they should spend it doing more. Keep a diary and write out the tasks to do, spreading them out over the week so that they do not bunch together. Ensure that every day there are breaks for rests and time alone. Having done all this and planned the week, stick to the plan! Try not to slip back into doing everything or feeling guilty about not doing more.

Setting limits: carers

1 Draw up a list of tasks that have to be done each week.
2 Plan in a diary when to do each task.
3 Make sure there are regular breaks.
4 Pace tasks: do not try to do everything at once.
5 Stick to your plan!

The other aspect of setting limits is dealing with demanding or unreasonable behaviour. This can be difficult, but a straight-forward approach is for the carer and injured person to set a number of practical ground rules and come to an agreement about what tasks the carer will do, and what the injured person has to deal with. One mother faced with unreasonable and unnecessary demands from her son for ·help with washing responded by coming to an agreement that she would do what was essential (in this case wash and dry his hair as he had difficulty lifting his arms above his head), but he had to do the rest. In short, she set a clear practical limit to her help, with the result that she had less to do and, equally importantly, helped her son to take more responsibility himself. It is important to set practical limits or targets like this, rather than something vague such as expecting the other person to be 'better behaved' or 'help more about the house'. Such targets are ill-defined and woolly, and it may not be at all clear if or when they have been achieved. Objective targets such as taking responsibility for the washing-up or hoovering are clear-cut, and everyone knows when they have been achieved and when they have not. It can be helpful to write down what has been agreed to overcome problems of forgetfulness and avoid disputes later. Finally, remember to stick to the agreement!

Sometimes head-injured people behave in ways that it would be desirable to help stop. Infantile or attention-seeking behav-iour are typical of such problems, as are rudeness or disinhibition. These behaviours can be difficult to discourage, and indeed the problem may lie in the fact that carers try to do so. Persuading, cajoling or reasoning with someone to stop them behaving a certain way may, in fact, act as a form of attention that ironically rewards or reinforces the behaviour. A much better strategy can be to pay the behaviour no attention at all and simply ignore it. Ignoring behaviour means that it is not rewarded and in time it is likely to disappear. One mother found her head-injured son's constant swearing, with frequent refer-ences to sex, extremely embarrassing and she repeatedly tried to discourage him to no effect. In fact he seemed perversely delighted by her discomfort and went out of his way to be rude when visitors were present. It seemed very likely that her reaction actually made matters worse, and so after a while she changed her approach and made no effort to discourage him at all. Whenever he swore she ignored him, no matter how embarrassed and tempted she was to say something. At first there was no change, but after a while the swearing became less frequent and he used less embarrassing swear-words. Ignoring undesirable behaviour can therefore be extremely effective, particularly if this approach is coupled by another strategy, which is to reward more desirable behaviour. To reduce disinhibited behaviour it may be best to ignore it and concentrate instead upon occasions when the person is behaving more appropriately, such as when working quietly or talking sensibly. In this way, the injured person gets the same amount of attention and interest, but only for appropriate conduct.

Setting limits: the injured relative
1   Agree who will do which tasks.
2   Be specific – identify practical goals and write them down.
3   Ignore inappropriate behaviour and encourage more appropriate behaviour.

Time alone
Many carers say that the most stressful aspect of looking after someone is that it is an unrelenting regime and they never have enough time for themselves. It is important for carers to set aside time, preferably every day, if only for half an hour. In addition, aim to go out alone one morning or afternoon and preferably for a whole day once a week. Relatives may be able to provide cover during that time, but if not the social services may arrange support. Carers should aim to take an annual holiday away from home; respite care may be arranged either through social services or charitable bodies. Many people feel guilty about leaving their relative and feel they are being 'selfish' in doing things for themselves. However, unless carers put time aside for rest, the strain may become so great that they are unable to provide the care they wish to provide. It is certainly not selfish for carers to consider their own needs and want to do things without their head-injured relative; it may give them the boost that is essential to help them cope.

Getting information
Most people are unfamiliar with what happens when someone has a head injury until it happens to them or someone they know. At first the changes can seem bizarre and frightening.

Inevitably there is a lot to learn and understand about both the medical and psychological effects, as well as practical matters such as benefit entitlements and what amenities are available locally. Good information is therefore essential and goes a long way towards making matters easier and more comprehensible. As carers discover, however, there are no proper statutory organisations in Britain where such information can easily be obtained, and they invariably find it difficult and frustrating getting information from hospital staff and other professionals. It therefore helps if carers are determined and become used to being persistent in getting what they want! Most people do not like to make a fuss and are intimidated by doctors, social workers, lawyers and other officials. However, to get the information and advice needed it is important not to keep quiet but be assertive and express concerns and queries. Most people need the help of several different professionals – GP, physiotherapist, social worker, psychologist – and it can therefore be useful to keep a notebook in which to record their names and addresses together with other useful information. Before seeing a new specialist, write out a list of questions and refer to it during the appointment. Jot down their answers during the appointment to avoid forgetting what was said. It is better to take notes than listen politely and then forget things later! If the advice is not clear, ask for an explanation: often the fault lies not with the carer but rather with the professional who has difficulty explaining issues in a straightforward way. If the answer or information is not satisfactory, it is important not to give up but go to another source. It is very unlikely that any one professional will know the answers to all the different queries carers and injured people have, so one should expect to have to ask several different people.

Support groups such as those organised by Headway (National Head Injuries Association) can be invaluable, not just for head-injured people but also for their carers, and partners and parents regularly attend most meetings. Talking to other parents or partners about their experiences can be one of the most useful ways of learning about head injury. People who have lived with a head-injured person are often much more knowledgeable on the subject than most professionals who may have little firsthand experience of what it is like.

Getting information

1 Before seeing a professional, write out a list of questions to ask.
2 Write down their answers.
3 Ask for an explanation if the advice was not clear.
4 Be prepared to see several professionals to get the information needed.
5 Join a support group and talk to other relatives of head-injured people – they are the best-informed.

7 Claiming compensation

For many people faced with the trauma of a head injury the last thing they think of is compensation and the law. Indeed, a large proportion of injured people fail to make a claim because they are unaware of their legal rights or they decide that they have no possibility of success. However, this is the wrong approach. Solicitors who specialise in accident work are often able to offer a first free interview to examine the prospects of a claim. A short interview with a specialist may open the door to substantial damages where previously it was thought there was no chance of redress.

Very often a head-injured person is assisted when conducting a claim by a 'next friend' or relative who liaises with the solicitors and barristers. A 'next friend' is appointed when the head-injured person is either below the age of eighteen or unable to manage his or her own affairs.

Naturally people are anxious about the prospect of a court hearing. However, in the vast majority of cases, claims are settled before the case ever gets to court and of those that actually get to the court doors, only a very small percentage are heard before a judge. Invariably an acceptable compromise is achieved to the satisfaction of all parties. The aim of the courts in awarding damages or compensation is, in financial terms, to put the injured person back to the position he or she was in before the injury. It is not commonly known, but claims are made up of different losses called 'heads of damage': damages are awarded for the actual injuries, loss of earnings (both past and future), the cost of care, and various other losses all of which are discussed in detail later. However, the maximum award for injury alone at present is only around £130,000. This stands in stark contrast to a claim for defamation of character, which resulted in awards of £500,000 to Jeffrey Archer or £1,000,000 to Elton John. Similarly, companies and individuals can be awarded millions of pounds in damages for economic loss. In the United States astronomic damages are awarded by the courts to injured persons. However, the UK courts are becoming more generous as specialist solicitors seek ways to increase the size of their clients' claims, and the development of what are called 'structured settlements' (which are discussed later) has opened up the possibility of substantial compensation to provide for the injured person throughout his or her life.

The selection and role of a solicitor

Where a person has been seriously injured it is vital that a specialist solicitor is selected by the claimant and his or her family. Such cases must be conducted by an expert and not by the claimant alone although, of course, he or she has every right to do so. Furthermore, the solicitor who is 'having a go' on his or her first case should be avoided. You may need to contact a number of solicitors and question them about their experience before you are satisfied that you have chosen the right solicitor for you. You can choose an appropriate solicitor by the following methods:

1 By contacting **National Headwa**y, which publishes (by region) a list of solicitors known to be experienced in this field.
2 You may then contact a **local Headway group** whose members may be able to answer any questions you have about local solicitors and guide you in the right direction.
3 **APIL (The Association of Personal Injury Lawyers)** is a new organisation of lawyers wholly committed to bringing claims on behalf of the injured. Again their database may be of use.
4 **The Law Society** can often recommend a number of solicitors in your area who can help. The Law Society has established a list of personal injury specialists which is available to the public.
5 **The local Citizens' Advice Bureau (CAB)** may be able to help, or the hospital social worker may have local knowledge of solicitors who practise in this area.

The addresses of these organisations are given at the end of this book.

Once you have selected a solicitor, do not be afraid to raise questions about his or her experience with your type of case.

Prepare for your interview by making notes of the questions that you feel are relevant. Also, make notes during the interview so that you can remember what you are told. You may want to ask the solicitor, for example, about the team he or she will put together, about costs, legal aid, the legal procedure and, of course, how long the litigation is likely to take. Experienced solicitors will not be offended by this: they will realise that there is a lot to take in all at once.

Do not delay in instructing a solicitor

The sooner a solicitor is instructed the quicker the claim will be resolved one way or the other. Often evidence needs to be gathered as soon as possible. Where, for example, someone is injured on a building site it may be essential that important evidence is speedily videotaped or photographed, owing to the changing nature of such a site. Similarly, because of the transient nature of the building trade, witnesses may need to be seen and interviewed before they become untraceable.

Another point to be aware of is that delay in bringing a claim can result in it being **time barred**. One generally has three years from the date of the injury to bring a claim, although the three-year rule does not apply to children until they reach the age of eighteen, after which the limitation clock starts to tick. People who are unable to manage their own affairs may also be unaffected by the limitation rule. In certain cases, the three-year period starts to run from the date the injured person knew that the injury was caused by a certain factor. Time limitation in many cases is decided by the courts, and in those cases expert advice is required from a solicitor and a barrister.

The role of a solicitor

Your solicitor should investigate the claim rapidly and gather the information required to prove the case in court. In particular he or she will collate the **evidence** required to prove fault on the part of another (this is called **liability**); secondly, he or she will investigate **causation**, in other words what caused the injury; thirdly, he or she will accumulate the evidence to prove all losses (**damages**) reasonably arising from the accident. In doing all of the above, it is your solicitor's duty to keep you regularly informed and get the claim to court as quickly as is reasonably possible.

The selection and role of a barrister

Through local knowledge you may have gathered that a particular barrister or Queen's Counsel specialises in head injury cases. Generally, however, you will rely upon the advice of your solicitor as to which barrister(s) to use. An experienced solicitor in this field will know at least a handful of Queen's Counsel (senior and more experienced barristers) who fit the bill. Queen's Counsel are referred to as 'QCs', 'leaders' or 'silks'. The particular experience of an individual QC might be appropriate in certain cases. For example, a certain Queen's Counsel might have a lot of experience in the medical negligence field, and your case might involve brain injury caused by oxygen starvation. Many barristers' chambers now publish a brochure which details the expertise of the barristers within the chambers. As a consequence, the range of expertise provided by the Bar is more widely known and understood. The best barristers are, of course, much in demand and have a heavy case-load, which may mean that they take some time to return papers to your solicitor. It may also be that you have to wait some time before you are able to see the barrister.

A barrister is trained to speak in court. He or she is an advocate and will know the judges, their natures, their moods and what they like and dislike. He or she will have the skill to present your case in the best possible light. In addition barristers advise clients 'in conference' (a meeting), provide written opinions on evidence and draft documents for the court. In serious cases a junior barrister will be used as well as a Queen's Counsel, although there has been a growing trend within the legal profession to authorise one barrister only in order to save costs.

Proving a claim to obtain compensation

The burden of proving fault lies with the person making the claim, who is called the claimant or **plaintiff**. The person or organisation who is sued (which is usually an insurance company) is called the **defendant**. The plaintiff has to show that the other party was **negligent** and that he or she owed the plaintiff a **duty of care**. In addition to convincing the judge that liability lies with the other party, the injured person has to show, by calling evidence, that the person at fault has breached his or her duty of care and fallen below the standard of care that one would normally expect. In a road traffic accident claim, for example, a person who goes through traffic lights while they show red and collides with a pedestrian lawfully crossing the road, owes that pedestrian a duty of care not to go through the red light. By going through the lights on red, the driver has fallen below the standard of care that one would expect of the ordinary, competent and prudent motorist. The driver would be found by the court to have been negligent.

In order to win any claim in the civil courts in the United Kingdom a claimant has to prove, **on the balance of probabilities**, that someone is liable; secondly, that the claimant has suffered loss, or will on the balance of probabilities suffer loss; and thirdly, that the loss was caused by the person liable. This evidential test must not be confused with the criminal burden of proof, namely that a case must be proved beyond reasonable doubt. Proving a case on the balance of probabilities is clearly a less demanding evidential burden.

Litigation, that is, suing for compensation, is tough, and the defendant or his or her insurers will try their level best to delay the claim and get away with paying nothing, or as little as possible. That is why it is vitally important to have an experienced solicitor acting for you, and the claim has to be pushed all the time to ensure a speedy conclusion. To do this a solicitor will have to investigate the three cardinal areas that are integral to your claim, namely **liability**, **causation** and **quantum** (damages).

Liability or fault

In order to prove that liability or fault lies with the defendant, your solicitor has to acquire **evidence** which can be presented to the trial judge, who then decides whether the defendant has a legal liability. If one takes a road accident as an example, your solicitor will need to obtain witness statements from yourself and others, photographs, perhaps even a video, a sketch plan or an engineer's report. He or she may have to make enquiries of the highway authority about the functioning of traffic signals. An accident reconstruction engineer may need to be employed to prepare mathematical calculations to show what probably happened in the vital seconds before the impact. Police officers may have to be interviewed. Your solicitor may have to attend the scene of the accident with witnesses so that they can make on-site statements as to what actually happened. Evidence must be collated at an early stage when the witnesses' memories are fresh.

Whether a claim arises out of a road traffic accident, a fall, a factory or industrial accident, or perhaps a case of medical negligence, one has to prove liability in order to establish fault. Once liability has been established, you can look at what loss has resulted from the negligent act (e.g., damages for injury and loss of income etc.). Before we cover this area, however, we should consider the situation in which the injured person might be found to be partially responsible for the accident. This is known as **contributory negligence**.

Contributory negligence

In some accidents the head-injured person may be found to have been partially responsible for what happened. A pedestrian may have attempted, for instance, to cross three lanes of a busy trunk road. An accident may have ensued in which he or she was struck by a vehicle while in the third lane, perhaps two or three paces from the kerb. The person might not have crossed at a nearby pelican crossing and in addition might have run across the road when it was dangerous to do so. Although in this sort of situation the driver of the vehicle should perhaps have seen the pedestrian and avoided a collision, the pedestrian might be partly to blame. As an example, the court could find the driver seventy-five per cent to blame and the pedestrian twenty-five per cent to blame. The pedestrian therefore would only recover seventy-five per cent of his or her damages. So if the damages were going to be £100,000, only £75,000 would be recovered because of the court's finding of contributory negligence. In most accidents insurers or defendants will try to find a way in which they can establish some form of contributory negligence. They will use all avenues to try and reduce any damages which are due to the injured plaintiff.

Causation

In many cases it will be clear that the injuries have been caused by, say, a car crash. However, matters could be clouded, for instance, if a person who is injured in a road traffic accident had been behaving in an unusual manner before the accident. In the course of surgery it may be found that the head-injured person had a large tumour on the brain. In these circumstances, the defendant's insurers might try to prove that the symptoms displayed by the injured person after the accident were not due to the head injury but to the tumour. This is a difficult question of causation on which expert medical opinion is necessary. In practice, however, causation is not normally such an issue in head injury cases, as it is often quite plain what caused the brain damage. In cases of medical negligence, particularly involving children who have suffered brain damage during birth, the issue of causation will be central: whether, for instance, it was the malpractice of the medical personnel or the position of the child during birth which caused the injury.

Quantum or damages

Once your solicitor has proven on the balance of probabilities that someone was negligent, he or she then has to prove, again on the balance of probabilities that you have suffered losses both in the past and future in order for you to be awarded compensation. In a head injury case there will be many different claims for compensation. The courts refer to these as **heads of damage**. As mentioned earlier, the court's objective in compensating somebody is to ensure that as far as possible they are restored to the same position, in financial terms, as they were in before the injury. Below are examples of the different types of heads of damage and the evidence that is required to support the claim. The list is not exhaustive but has been prepared to give you some idea of the sort of work your solicitor has to undertake to prove your losses to the defendants and the court.

1 **General damages for pain, suffering and loss of amenity**. This is the award given to compensate for the actual injuries suffered. The awards are pitifully low, the highest most recent award being a figure of just over £130,000. This appears to be the current ceiling, although solicitors and barristers are always trying to increase this head of damage. In cases of the utmost severity this award very often reflects a mere ten per cent of the total damages. In order to prove this head of damage, evidence is required. Reports from a consultant neurologist and a consultant neuropsychologist are essential in head injury cases. Perhaps two or three reports

will be required from each expert throughout the course of the case. Additional reports in particular cases may also be required from other experts. The defendant's solicitors will, in all probability, wish to have the claimant examined by their own expert neurologist and neuropsychologist. If the claimant fails to co-operate in being examined by these specialists, the defendant's solicitors are entitled to apply to the court to have the action 'stayed'. This means that a court order is granted to the defendant's solicitors preventing the case from proceeding further until the claimant has been examined by their experts. It is therefore important to co-operate with the defendant's solicitors' requests for examinations.

2 **Interest on general damages for pain, suffering and loss of amenity**. Interest on general damages is awarded at the rate of two per cent from the date of service of the proceedings on the defendant. This is the reason why it is important to get proceedings instigated as soon as reasonably possible. Three years' interest on a sum of £120,000 is £6,600. A solicitor who drags his or her feet with the action, and fails or is slow to serve proceedings, is potentially negligent and could cost his or her client sizeable sums of money. Likewise, a person who is slow to instruct a solicitor is losing money by delay.

3 **Damages for loss of past earnings**. Here evidence is obtained from employers or accountants as to the actual losses sustained up to the date of settlement of the claim or the trial of the claim. If someone has an intermittent history of pre-accident employment the matter becomes somewhat complicated. A work history will have to be obtained from the claimant, and perhaps the assistance of an employment specialist who will refer to local and national employment statistics to help prove this head of claim.

4 **Tangible losses**. Examples of tangible losses would be a claim for a motor vehicle or for clothing damaged in the accident.

5 **Travelling expenses**. The expenses of the family and claimant in travelling to and from hospital for appointments can add up to quite a sizeable sum. A diary should be kept by the family to record details of all trips, so that a proper claim for damages can be prepared.

6 **Loss of a company car**. This can sometimes be a very relevant loss, particularly as so many people in this country are provided with a company vehicle. The claim is calculated from the date of the injury, and will include a future claim for loss of the company vehicle if it can be shown that the claimant will not work again and, but for the injury, would have been provided with a company vehicle until the date of retirement.

7 **Past care**. In most cases, a great deal of care is provided by the head-injured person's family and friends. The family should keep a diary of all the effort and care that has been provided from the date of the injury. This will prove invaluable to the solicitor when calculating the cost of care provided up to the date of settlement or trial. It can also be a useful guide as to the amount of care likely to be needed in the future. Basically, this claim is calculated by finding out the number of hours which have been expended by the carer over and above that which would normally be provided but for the head injury. For each hour expended, a sum of money is notionally allocated and calculated thereafter on an annual basis. Quite considerable sums of money can be awarded for both past and future care.

To assist in the calculation of the amount of care which is likely to be provided, the services of an occupational therapist and a nursing expert are usually engaged. The defendant's solicitors may wish to use their own care expert or nursing specialist, who will prepare a report for their benefit. Again, the claimant must co-operate if the defendant wishes to have his or her expert complete an assessment. If the defendants intend to rely upon their care report, they must release a copy to the claimant's solicitors, otherwise they are debarred from using it. Generally, a copy of the other side's report is never produced if it does not challenge the calculations made in the claimant's expert's report.

8 Interest can be recovered on items of expenditure which do not involve a continuing loss (e.g., a written-off motor vehicle). Where losses are continuous up to the date of settlement (e.g., loss of earnings) interest is available at half the usual rate.

9 **Damages for the partial cost of new accommodation**. A head-injured person may sometimes be so disabled that

new premises specifically designed for his or her needs are required. Architectural evidence may be obtained from an expert in the form of a report. Certain accommodation costs can be included as part of the claim.

10 **Future losses**. This can include damages for loss of future earnings, damages for the cost of future care, damages for loss of pension rights and damages for future loss of congenial employment.

Future losses are calculated by what solicitors call the **multiplier** and **multiplicand** system. In the case of a 21-year-old man who was earning £10,000 net per annum, this figure would be the multiplicand. He might have worked until he was sixty-five years old were it not for the injury. You might say that he is therefore entitled to forty-four years' loss of earnings. Unfortunately it does not work like that. The maximum judicial multiplier for loss of earnings which the courts will apply is seventeen years' loss (that is, the multiplier is at most seventeen). Thus 17 x £10,000 = £170,000 for loss of future earnings. The multiplier decreases as the claimant's age increases. The logic for the low multiplier is that the young man here is recovering compensation now and is able to invest that sum so that it will provide him with an income equal to that which he would have earned but for the accident. Needless to say, the income needs to be invested wisely in order to achieve that ideal. The multiplier and multiplicand system is applied to most future loss claims.

The use of a specialist centre

Where means permit, it is often beneficial for a head-injured person to attend a specialist head injury centre. Such centres are usually in the private sector, and to gain a place the defendant's insurers have to be persuaded to pay the cost of treatment. Head injury centres provide a range of therapies, including occupational therapy, physiotherapy, speech therapy and psychological input, and significant improvements can be obtained for those fortunate enough to have had the benefit of treatment. Often such centres also provide a report and video for the court. A case management system can also sometimes be provided to assist with the reintegration of the head-injured person into the community. The case management system involves a chosen individual looking after the needs of the injured person, assisting and guiding him or her in the daily chores of living, and is initiated when the person leaves the unit.

A 'day-in-the-life' video

Judges and insurers are able to get a clearer picture of a person's future and daily needs by seeing one of these videos. The videos record a typical day in the life of a head-injured person from getting up to going to bed, perhaps also showing any difficulties encountered at night. Again, this specialist evidence is very helpful to a judge when trying to assess the proper damages which should be awarded.

The risks of litigation

In litigation things can go horribly wrong in the witness box, and a judge might prefer one person's evidence to another's; or the judge might not be as generous in assessing damages as one might have hoped. It is for this reason that towards the conclusion of a case you might hear talk of a discount to the claim by perhaps as much as fifteen per cent for 'the risks of litigation'. What this means is that the defendant's solicitors offer you less money to settle out of court. In these circumstances you need clear, understandable advice from your legal adviser. Fifteen per cent of a claim worth £1,000,000 is £150,000, which may well be worth fighting for. The 'discount for the risks of litigation' is something which you come across in practice but is not often mentioned in textbooks.

The court system through to hearing

Accident claims are brought in the civil courts, not the criminal courts. The civil courts are perhaps not as awesome as the criminal courts to those who are not familiar with the court system. The civil courts have to decide whether compensation is payable rather than whether a person is guilty or not guilty. A single judge will hear the evidence for the plaintiff and the defendant and afterwards will deliver his or her judgement, which is sometimes delayed to another day in a particularly difficult or lengthy case. A claim is usually initiated in the local County court if it is worth less than £50,000. If a case is worth more than £50,000 an action will be commenced in the High Court. Most head injury claims are brought in the High Court.

In both High Court and County court claims, the court requires solicitors to prepare pleadings. The pleadings state in written form what the issues are between the parties. Thus, when a judge comes to hear the case, he or she can read the pleadings before coming into court and know why the plaintiff holds the defendant responsible for the accident and what compensation he or she is claiming. Similarly, the judge can immediately see if the action is defended, and why the defendant says he or she is not responsible or only partly responsible for the accident.

Payments into court

This is arguably the strongest weapon which a defendant's insurers have in their armoury. A payment into court can be a very tempting and persuasive method of preventing a claim going to court and occurs when the defendant's solicitors pay into court a sum of money which they say satisfies all the claims made by the plaintiff. Once such a payment has been made the money can either be accepted or rejected. A payment into court is not in itself an admission of fault on the part of the defendant; it might be economically advisable to make such a payment rather than let the case go to trial. Many claimants, however, interpret a payment as a form of admission of fault.

Once the payment has been made, you will generally have twenty-one days in which to decide whether to accept or reject it. Once accepted, the money is paid to your solicitors within a matter of weeks. However, following consultation with your solicitor, and in some cases your barrister, you may decide to reject the payment. In advising you, your solicitor will take into account the prospect of complete or partial success of your claim, and the amount of compensation you might expect to receive. If a decision is made to reject the payment a number of possibilities arise:

1 The defendant could make a further payment into court increasing the amount. In this case a further twenty-one days for acceptance or rejection would come into operation.

2 The defendant could make what is known as a 'without

prejudice offer' to pay more than the money presently in court and try to settle the claim by negotiation. Again, your solicitor will advise you appropriately should this occur.

3 The defendant may indicate that they are not prepared to increase the payment into court and the matter will then have to proceed to trial. Although defendants give this indication, they may sometimes still come forward with further offers, even on the day of the court hearing.

It is important to understand the consequences of rejection of the payment into court. If the matter proceeds to trial the judge hearing the case knows nothing about it. He or she will hear the evidence and make a decision as to where responsibility lies and whether any degree of blame attaches to you. Having reached the decision about responsibility, the judge will then assess the amount of compensation. At that point, he or she will be informed that a payment into court has been made. If you are subsequently awarded more money than has been paid into court, then you have effectively won the case. You will receive the compensation awarded by the judge and the defendant will be responsible for your legal costs and expenses (the question of costs is discussed later). However, should the judge award the same or less money than was paid into court, then he or she will order that you must pay all your legal costs and all the defendant's expenses from the date the payment into court was made. The defendant will still be responsible for the costs before that date, but it is almost always the case that the most expensive part of an action will be after the payment into court: particularly at the trial, where the attendance of solicitors and barristers, medical and other expert witnesses, as well as lay witnesses all have to be paid for. In such circumstances, the costs that fall upon you will be substantial and may drastically reduce the amount of compensation you eventually receive. In extreme cases, it may mean that you receive no compensation and still have a liability for costs.

Many people feel that the rules regarding payments into court provide defendants with some sort of unfair advantage. The rationale behind the rules is to enable defendants to deal with claims that are unnecessarily taken to full court hearings, and, where a reasonable settlement could be reached, without the costs of a full hearing.

The trial or hearing

This is clearly a nerve-racking day for the plaintiff and his or her family. There may have been a payment into court which has been rejected, and the plaintiff is now faced with reliving the accident and facing the trauma of a day or days in court. As the court is an alien place to most people, the whole experience can be very intimidating.

On the day of the hearing there will be meetings between clients and solicitors. Many people will be walking around the court corridors in black gowns and wigs. People will be scurrying in and out of interview rooms and having discussions about the cases that are proceeding. There will be last-minute discussions between all parties, and perhaps offers and counter-offers of settlement. Witnesses who have attended the hearing to give evidence might on the day, by some miracle, have had their evidence agreed by the objecting party. The atmosphere is often frenetic, principally because the judge quite properly wants to start his or her list of hearings promptly.

Cases are often capable of agreement at the court doors. This usually happens because all the people who matter are at court at the same time, and decisions can be made there and then as a result of legal advice given.

In head injury cases, there will almost inevitably have been a meeting or conference between the client and the barristers before the trial where all the issues concerning liability, causation and quantum will have been aired and digested. If the case is incapable of settlement, it will proceed to trial. When this happens, the plaintiff's barrister will open the case by explaining to the judge what the claim is about and the issues of fact and law on which he or she will be asked to decide.

The barrister for the plaintiff will then ask the witnesses for the plaintiff to give evidence in turn. Each witness will give his or her evidence and be asked questions by the plaintiff's barrister. This is known as 'examination-in-chief'. Once the examination-in-chief has been concluded, the barrister for the defendant will ask the witnesses questions resulting from their earlier evidence. This is known as 'cross-examination'. In cross-examining a witness, the barrister has the opportunity of asking searching questions and, of course, he or she can ask leading questions. A leading question is one which might lead the witness to provide a certain answer, such as 'John Smith caused the accident by crashing into the vehicle, didn't he?'. Here the answer is included in the question.

Unless witnesses are deemed by the court to be experts they are only entitled to give evidence of fact and hearsay evidence is generally not allowed. Generally speaking, the courts are only interested in what you as a witness saw, not what somebody else told you they saw, which is perhaps a simple explanation of hearsay evidence in its most general form.

Expert witnesses (e.g., doctors, engineers etc.) will then be called to give evidence. Expert witnesses are empowered by law to give expert opinions upon which the trial judge can place as much reliance as he or she deems appropriate. Expert witnesses are subject to examination-in-chief and cross-examination just like other witnesses. Once all the plaintiff's witnesses have been heard, the defendant's barrister calls all his or her witnesses into the witness box. They in turn are subject to the rules governing examination-in-chief, cross-examination, expert opinion evidence and, of course, hearsay. Once all the evidence has been heard by the judge, he or she will listen to the closing speeches made by the barristers for the plaintiff and defendant. The judge then has the task of giving judgement on the issues that were presented before the court. When delivered, the judgement is binding on all parties to the action.

Funding the claim

The initial interview
Specialist solicitors are often prepared to give a first free interview to a potential claimant. Solicitors who specialise in this field may have disabled facilities with ground-floor interview rooms, although if you are unable to get to the solicitor's office he or she will often come to see you either in hospital or at home. In serious cases many solicitors are prepared to travel the country to obtain new clients.

Legal aid
The Legal Aid Board grants franchises to certain solicitors which mean that they are given certain powers by the Legal Aid Board. Such solicitors are judged to be proficient in the admin-

istration and handling of Legal Aid claims. However, some firms with similar experience of Legal Aid work will, for their own reasons, have chosen not to apply for a franchise. They should, however, be just as able to conduct a Legal Aid claim as a firm which has a franchise.

1 Your solicitor will provide and assist you with the completion of Legal Aid forms and supply you with information leaflets. He or she will advise you how the scheme works and explain about the Legal Aid Board's **statutory charge** (which is explained later on in this section). This relates to the claim which the Legal Aid Board has on damages in certain circumstances, when your solicitor's legal expenses are not fully recovered from the losing party.

2 Since 1990 children have been able to qualify for Legal Aid without reference to their parents' financial resources. This means that in the majority of cases children will qualify for Legal Aid, provided the Legal Aid Board is satisfied that the case requires investigation with the support of public funds.

3 In certain cases the solicitor will advise you initially under the Legal Aid Board **Green Form scheme**. This pays for two hours' advice by the solicitor. Unfortunately the number of people who are financially eligible for this advice has been dramatically reduced in the last ten years.

4 Your solicitor will submit the completed forms to your local Legal Aid Area Office. The time for processing a claim can vary from office to office. People who receive Income Support will generally receive an offer more quickly than someone who has to submit his or her last three years' audited accounts. For those who are not in receipt of Income Support, a further questionnaire will be forwarded by the relevant DSS office in connection with income, capital, and expenditure. The sooner the forms are returned the sooner the Legal Aid will be determined. With your consent, some solicitors will start work on the claim whilst they are awaiting the decision on Legal Aid. Others prefer to wait until the Legal Aid Certificate has been granted, which, when issued, guarantees payment to the solicitor for work undertaken.

5 You may have to pay a monthly **contribution** towards your Legal Aid. The contribution is returnable, although without any interest, upon the successful completion of the case, provided there is no claim for legal fees on the Legal Aid

Fund. It follows therefore that the quicker the claim is concluded, the fewer the number of contributions which have to be paid.

6 When a person is legally aided the Legal Aid Board agrees to pay any reasonably incurred legal fees. Where damages are recovered, the Legal Aid Board has a first claim on the damages until the legally aided person subsequently recovers all his or her legal costs from the losing party, or the insurers. This means that in some, but not all, circumstances there can be a delay between the date when damages are recovered to the date when they are actually paid to the claimant.

7 Once a Legal Aid Certificate is issued it will either have no **limitation** endorsed, or the Legal Aid Board will impose a limitation on the work which your solicitors may do within the Legal Aid scheme. For example, in a road accident the solicitor's role may be restricted to obtaining a police report, or in a medical negligence claim he or she may be limited to obtaining the complete medical records and then getting an expert's written opinion. Similarly, in an industrial accident your solicitors might only be allowed to obtain a consulting engineer's report. The Legal Aid Certificate may be limited particularly when the issue of liability (fault) is unclear. In this cost-conscious society the Legal Aid Board has now also started to restrict the amount of money which can be spent on a case. Once that limit has been reached, permission is needed from the Legal Aid Board to proceed further.

8 Your case might be held up as a solicitor will be obliged to obtain **prior authority** from the Legal Aid Board to incur certain expenditure (e.g., to instruct a Queen's Counsel, arrange a brain scan, or prepare a video). Until that expenditure is authorised the expert cannot undertake such work.

9 If you fail to maintain any of the monthly contributions or have been advised by your solicitors that your case is unlikely to succeed, your Legal Aid Certificate may well be discharged (that is to say, cancelled). This means that your solicitor is no longer authorised to do any more work for you under the Legal Aid scheme. Payment for any work done thereafter, including letters, telephone calls and meetings, will be your responsibility. If you have not recovered costs

from the other party the contributions you have paid to the Legal Aid Fund will be used to pay your own legal fees. If the legal fees are less than your contributions there will be a refund to you of the balance. However, in most cases contributions will be swallowed up by the costs, as cases of the utmost severity are not cheap to fund. In addition, no interest is returned.

Union backing

If you are a member of a union the terms of membership very often allow your union to fund your legal fees. This can be particularly relevant in industrial injury cases. The choice of solicitor is, however, usually restricted to those firms which have close links with the unions.

Legal expenses insurance

If you have purchased a legal expenses insurance policy before the accident, your legal fees may be covered to allow you to bring a claim. Freedom in choosing a solicitor can, however, be restricted to a panel solicitor.

Interim payments

Some people are not eligible for Legal Aid, and nor do they have any other means to fund a case. An interim payment can often be obtained from the defendants when it is clear that the claimant will recover damages once the case is concluded. An interim payment can then be used to pay the various experts to provide reports which are essential to the successful conclusion of the case. In addition to paying experts' fees, they can also be used to fund the cost of private rehabilitation at a specialist head injury unit or to purchase specialist accommodation. An interim payment can either be made voluntarily by the paying party or obtained through the courts. The rule affecting interim payments is that in the event of no damages being recovered, or the damages recovered being less than the interim payment received, the balance or whole of the interim payment is repayable.

Private means

If you are unable to obtain any of the above methods of funding, you will be obliged to fund the case out of your own pocket.

Solicitors are required to inform their clients regularly about fees and make charges every three months so that the plaintiff knows exactly where he or she stands as to the costs of the case. When a client is paying the solicitor privately, the hourly rate charged might be different from that allowed by the Legal Aid Board or the courts. Despite Law Society regulations to the contrary, many solicitors will charge out of the damages recovered and bill the client at the end of the case rather than from the beginning. A client who funds a case privately is exposed financially. If the case is lost, the client is responsible for the costs not only of his or her own legal advisers but also for the legal costs of the person he or she has sued.

Costs and solicitors' charges

If you are funding a claim from your own resources you will have to pay your solicitor an agreed hourly rate. This could vary considerably depending on the complexity of the case, whom you choose and where your solicitor is situated. An experienced solicitor in the City in London, with higher overheads, will charge much more than a similarly experienced solicitor in the provinces. In addition, the solicitor will charge approximately one tenth of the hourly rate for each telephone call and letter. It therefore pays to shop around if you are funding a claim yourself. If you win your case your legal costs will, of course, be recovered either partially or wholly from the losing party but there might be a shortfall which could mean that you have to pay your solicitor's costs out of your damages.

Fees are often charged by others to your solicitor and have to be paid by him or her. These are called disbursements. These include, for example, barristers' fees, doctors' fees, care specialists' fees, police report fees and engineers' fees, to name but a few. If you are funding the case yourself, your solicitor will usually ask for these sums in advance, so that he or she is in credit when the time comes to pay the bill.

In the British courts the party which loses the civil action generally pays the winning party's 'reasonable costs'. In the event of a dispute 'reasonable costs' are adjudicated by the court, which will look at the winning party's bill of costs and decide exactly how much the loser has to pay. In this situation it is possible that the winning party might recover, say, £100 for each hour worked by his or her solicitor. However, if the winning party has agreed with his or her solicitor (in non-Legal Aid cases) to pay £120 per hour, he or she will be liable for that shortfall, unless the court orders otherwise.

What happens at the end of the case?

Winning the case

If you win your case and you are legally aided, your solicitor is obliged to pay all your damages into the Legal Aid Fund where the money will earn interest until his or her costs have been agreed and paid by the losing party. There is an exception to this rule: in certain circumstances your solicitor can pay you some of your damages on account pending the finalisation of his or her fees. Once the solicitor's fees have been agreed, provided the Legal Aid Board does not have to pay any of the fees, you will receive the balance of your damages. If, however, the Legal Aid Board has to pay a proportion of your solicitor's fees, you may then lose that proportion of your damages and/or contribution paid – in other words the Legal Aid Board Statutory Charge attaches to that proportion of your damages/contribution. It has to be said that in a large proportion of cases the successful claimant who is legally aided will recover payment of all his or her legal expenses. If you have paid a contribution towards your Legal Aid this will be returned to you, although unfortunately without any interest being paid.

Losing the case

Clearly, we all hope that this does not happen. Statistics show that over ninety per cent of people who are involved in personal injury cases successfully conclude their cases by recovering damages. The general rule of 'loser pays costs' does not in most cases apply to legally aided claimants. Usually costs which have been awarded against the legally aided party are not enforced without the 'leave of the court'. This means that you do not have to pay the successful defendant's costs unless the court orders it. In the majority of cases that is the end of the matter. Where a legally aided litigant has paid no contribution towards his or her Legal Aid there will be nothing further to pay. Where, however, a contribution has been paid, this will be used by the Legal Aid Board as part payment towards solicitors' fees. In this situation, the Statutory Charge applies to any money which you have paid towards your Legal Aid.

If there has been a payment into court and the judge awards less than that figure, there is a serious risk that any damages recovered will be used primarily to pay the defendant's costs from the date of the payment into court, as well as your solicitor's legal fees from the date of the payment into court. Here a sizeable chunk of your damages could be utilised to pay the costs incurred after the date of the payment into court.

The taxation procedure

If, upon winning your case, your solicitor is unable to agree with the opposing solicitors any part of his or her professional fees, the matter usually proceeds to what is called 'taxation'. Taxation, unfortunately, causes delay. First of all, your solicitor has to prepare a bill of costs. This can take some considerable time, as he or she has to itemise each letter, telephone call and meeting and describe in detail all the work that has been done. In a lengthy case this can take weeks to prepare. The bill is then lodged at the court and a District Judge reviews the bill and listens to any objections made by the paying party as well as any representations made by your solicitor. You too might need to attend this hearing, because if you are legally aided you might be obliged to pay some of your solicitor's bill if some of the costs are awarded against the Legal Aid Fund. In those circumstances, as stated above, the Statutory Charge attaches to your damages.

It can take anything up to a year or even longer after your case has been concluded for the taxation procedure to be completed. This is frustrating for you because some of your damages will be held back until then. It is also frustrating for your solicitor because he or she will have to wait to be paid (remember he or she may have spent several years getting the case to court). A new system of taxation is imminent: time will show whether it is an improvement on the old one.

Infants, persons with a disability and the Court of Protection

Infants

Once a claim has been concluded either after a trial or settlement, and a sum of money has been agreed to be paid to a child, a hearing will be convened to enable the court to lend its approval to the settlement. At that hearing, which is usually heard in chambers and not in open court, the judge will listen to the representations made on behalf of the plaintiff and the defendant. He or she will read the relevant evidence on liability, causation and quantum and decide whether he or she feels the agreed figure is acceptable. The infant and parent or next friend will be obliged to attend the hearing and answer any questions raised by the judge. If the judge is satisfied, he or she will approve the settlement which then becomes an order of the court.

Compensation is then usually invested by the court at the Public Trust Office in London, where it is managed and invested until the child is eighteen years of age, after which all of the fund is payable to him or her. At the age of eighteen, the plaintiff goes to the court with a copy of the court order, his or her birth certificate and proof of identification and the court will then arrange for payment.

Persons with a disability or 'patients'

Most head-injured people can manage their affairs quite satisfactorily, but there are those who are unable to do so. Often the advice of a consultant neurologist will be sought if there is any doubt. If the plaintiff is considered unable to manage his or her own affairs an application will be made to the Court of Protection to appoint a receiver. The Court of Protection is a section of the High Court based in London which manages the finances of those unable to look after their affairs.

Professional advisors are empowered by the Court of Protection to invest the sum of money awarded and an annual administrative charge is deducted from the income generated. A member of the family is usually appointed as receiver, which means that he or she deals with the day-to-day financial affairs of the plaintiff and applies to the court when further sums of money are required. The Court of Protection, as its name implies, protects the disabled person from unscrupulous people who, given the opportunity, would take advantage of him or her. The Court of Protection will manage the affairs of the 'patient' until he or she dies, whereupon any balance of capital and income forms part of the person's estate.

Structured settlements

Before the introduction of structured settlements in the United Kingdom in 1989, all large injury damage claims were settled by way of the conventional lump sum award. Recently structured settlements have attracted a good deal of media coverage due to the impressive figures that can be earned by an injured person. Essentially, every solicitor advising an injured plaintiff should explore the possibility of making a structured settlement. Failure to do so could result in the solicitor being found negligent in law!

What are structured settlements and how do they work?

There is a view that a structured settlement should be considered for any award exceeding £50,000. Before a judgement is obtained, the claim is quantified under the conventional award system and a final figure is agreed between the parties. With a portion of those damages, the defendant's insurer then purchases what is called an annuity (or annuities) from a life office assurance company. There are therefore two contracts: one that the plaintiff has with the insurer to pay him or her an annual sum; and a contract that the insurer has with the life office assurance company. The plaintiff usually keeps some of the compensation as a 'contingency fund' for any major items of expenditure (such as a house or car), that might be required in the future. The plaintiff is then paid a sum of money every year by the insurer.

Advantages and disadvantages of a structured settlement

Structured settlements are tax-free and usually index-linked and the income can be guaranteed for a minimum number of years. One can have more than one annuity which start to provide additional income at significant financial points in the injured person's future years. This is particularly useful when it is anticipated that there will be increased costs of care some time in the future. A further advantage is that if there is a disagreement between the plaintiff and defendant, say, on liability and quantum, a structure may bridge the gap and help achieve a settlement. Finally, a structured settlement prevents a frivolous plaintiff from dissipating a large sum which is supposed to last for life.

One of the disadvantages of a structured settlement is that the whole of the plaintiff's damages are not within his or her control. In addition, if the insurer subsequently becomes insolvent, the plaintiff cannot recover the annual payment. Solicitors should consider this possibility before agreeing to a structure and should insure against this risk. The lump sum award avoids the risk of the insurance company becoming insolvent. There is also a certain degree of finality for the defendant's insurer with a lump sum settlement, which is attractive: the case is finished and off the books. With a structured settlement, the insurer has to have administrative staff to liaise with the life office, the Inland Revenue and the plaintiff for many years to come. Some insurers therefore shy away from structured settlements, and as there is no legal obligation on them to enter into one, that is the end of the matter. Finally, once established, structured settlements are inflexible. The annual sum cannot be altered. The plaintiff will, however, in certain cases, have the contingency lump sum fund to draw upon for any unusual items of future capital expenditure.

Availability of the structured settlement

Structured settlements are generally available to all plaintiffs ranging from a brain-damaged infant to an adult who is unable to manage his or her affairs. However, cases where the defendants are the Criminal Injuries Compensation Board (CICB) and the Motor Insurers' Bureau (MIB) are not eligible for a structured settlement. In addition, some local authorities that self-insure cannot make structured settlements. However, health authorities are now able to structure claims for damages made against them. Structured settlements are still available even when the plaintiff is partly responsible for the accident.

8 Looking to the future

Once the immediate shock of the accident or fall has passed, relatives and head-injured people want to know how much recovery is likely to occur, how long it will take, and what the future holds. These are difficult questions to answer because the effects of brain trauma vary enormously from one person to another, and while there are guidelines there are no hard and fast answers. Every doctor knows of patients who have had horrendous injuries – and it may even have been touch and go whether they would survive – and yet a year later they were coping apparently satisfactorily with their lives. Others sustain what appear to be far less serious injuries and yet never seem to recover sufficiently to resume their usual routine and cope with work. Such examples only go to show the complex effects of damage to the brain and how people respond to their injuries. Nevertheless we shall consider each of these questions in turn to see what general answers can be given, bearing in mind that these guidelines will not always apply to everyone.

How much recovery is likely?

In the days and weeks after brain trauma it is not always possible to predict with confidence what the eventual outcome is likely to be, and the most straightforward answer a doctor can give is that he or she simply does not know. Several factors influence recovery, including the person's age, his or her state of health before the injury, the severity of the trauma, and the development of early complications. As regards age, a far higher proportion of adults than children die following a severe head injury, and fewer adults attain a good recovery. This may reflect the younger brain's greater flexibility in the face of trauma, or it may be due to additional health problems in adults, who may smoke and drink alcohol excessively.

The severity of the head injury is obviously an important

factor in determining the outcome. There is a relationship between initial scores on the Glasgow Coma Scale (which was discussed in chapter 2) and a person's eventual recovery: the lower the coma score the worse the long-term outcome. For instance, the majority of people who are in a coma for more than two months die, and most of the remainder are left severely disabled; that is, they are dependent on others for daily support. On the other hand, those with mild head injuries (defined by a Glasgow Coma Scale score of between thirteen and fifteen) in the main return to their normal lifestyles.

When assessing outcome after head injury the first difficulty is deciding how to measure it. To someone with a mild head injury persisting memory problems may appear a real problem, whereas someone who has had a severe injury might wish that was their only complaint. Equally a mild loss of dexterity in the left hand may be an insignificant problem to a labourer, while to a pianist it would be a disaster. Broadly speaking, however, it is possible to classify outcomes after a head injury into three broad groups (leaving aside death and the persistent vegetative state). This classification constitutes what is called the Glasgow Outcome Scale which is often used by doctors to rate a person's level of recovery.

- **Severe disability** refers to those who are conscious but dependent on others for daily support by reason of mental or physical disability, or both. Depending on resources and the degree of family support, a proportion of people in this group will be institutionalised.
- **Moderate disability** indicates independence in daily activities, such as using public transport. Despite residual problems, for example, limb weakness, impairment of memory or personality change, people in this group are able to work in a sheltered environment.
- **Good recovery** implies return to a normal lifestyle even though there may be minor physical or psychological problems. Such people are fit to pursue their normal occupation.

The Glasgow Outcome Scale parallels the Glasgow Coma Scale (GCS), so that a low GCS score after a head injury often predicts a poor outcome.

While these and other such guidelines exist, it is nevertheless difficult for doctors to predict for each individual precisely what the future will bring. Part of the difficulty about giving a definite opinion is that, as we have seen, head injury can bring about a range of problems – medical, cognitive, temperamental and behavioural – and recovery does not always take place in these different areas at the same rate or to the same degree. Some people make a good medical recovery and have few or no lasting physical complaints, yet have suffered psychological changes (such as loss of memory) and personality changes which are quite disabling. Others have predominantly physical problems, such as difficulty walking, while from the psychological perspective they may be relatively unaffected. Unfortunately it is difficult to predict how much recovery is likely to take place in each of these different areas, and when pressed most doctors only feel able to give an uncertain and qualified reply. This can be hard to accept, and the honest answer 'wait and see' may not be satisfactory at a time when patient and family feel they need certainty. Anything more definite, however, whether optimistic or pessimistic, may be misleading.

How long will recovery take?

This is also a difficult question to answer in a straightforward way because each individual is different and has a range of problems particular to him or her. Different problems are resolved at different rates: for instance, a person may make good progress recovering from his or her physical injuries but far slower progress in overcoming forgetfulness or distractibility. Recovery relating to physical problems clearly depends on the precise nature of the bodily injuries sustained; some people may be relatively unscathed, whereas others may have extensive injuries, in addition to brain damage, which necessitate a long period of hospital care and rehabilitation. Psychological recovery occurs at different rates in different people. Research studies which have involved testing the intelligence of head-injured people and assessing their memory suggest that the first year after the injury is an extremely important period and a great deal of the total improvement takes place during that time. Worthwhile recovery may, however, continue into the second year, and sometimes there may even be further slight improvements after that. There are, however, wide differences between individuals and, for some, most recovery in their cognitive abilities takes place in the first year and there is little change thereafter; whereas others continue to improve at a much slower rate. It is important to bear in mind that our understanding of the pattern of recovery has in the main been derived from research studies of people who received little or no specialised rehabilitation for their psychological problems. In Britain this applies to the majority of head-injured people. However, developments in designing and implementing psychological treatments for problems such as forgetfulness and impaired attention hold the promise of a far different pattern of recovery in the future. As we have seen in the preceding chapters, there are also many practical steps that can be taken to alleviate problems, and it would be wrong to conclude that just because a certain interval of time has elapsed nothing more can be done. Memory aids, mnemonic strategies, a structured routine and other techniques may help overcome cognitive problems, while activity, challenging negative thinking and relaxation techniques can lessen emotional problems.

What does the future hold?

Over ninety per cent of people who have a head injury resume the activities and interests they had prior to the trauma, and only a minority suffer from continuing disability. If a person has cognitive and emotional problems, what happens to them in the long term? As we know, once the brain is damaged it cannot be repaired medically and therefore the damage is permanent. Research studies of people who have had severe head injuries suggest that in the long term the emotional and cognitive problems persist. One study in Scotland looked at a group of people with severe head injuries five years after they sustained their injuries and found that the psychological and behavioural problems were still present; in some cases they had even got worse. Relatives found the strain of caring considerable and this was mainly due to having to cope with these psychological problems. In short, research studies tend to come to the rather pessimistic conclusion that after severe head injury psychological problems do not gradually improve. If behavioural problems worsen this is unlikely to be due to a deterioration in the person's neurological condition, but rather because they become frustrated, angry and depressed and react to their circumstances. Once again, however, it is important to point out that our understanding of the long-term effects of head injury is derived in the main from studies of people who received minimal or no continuing long-term care once their immediate hospital treatment had finished; it may well be that developments in the rehabilitation and treatment of head injuries will mean that the future for head-injured people will be very different.

Returning to work

Getting back to work is an important goal for most people. Work, of course, brings an income, but also, and often more importantly, it allows independence and the achievement of personal goals, as well as a feeling of making progress and being successful. It also provides the opportunity to meet people and often a social life, and at a basic level it brings structure to the day. Deprived of these things, most people, whether or not they have had a head injury, begin to be depressed and despondent and feel that their life lacks purpose. Brain trauma is particularly likely to result in time off work, and unemployment, at least for a while, is not uncommon. One study found that the employment rate of a sample of severely head-injured people fell from eighty-six per cent before their injuries to twenty-nine per cent afterwards. Furthermore, five years after their injury seventy per cent of the group had still not managed to get back to work and remained unemployed. Whether or not a person gets back to work depends, of course, on many different factors. The economic climate, both locally and nationally, is clearly likely to be crucial, and at a time of recession it may be extremely difficult for a person with a disability to find work. However, there are many other factors which play a role in determining whether employment is achievable. Research studies suggest that young head-injured people are more likely to find work than those who are middle-aged or older, and those who had managerial jobs or work of a technical nature may also be more likely to resume their jobs. The presence of cognitive and personality problems has a very significant influence on whether work is possible. This is not surprising: employers often have little understanding or experience of head injury, and they may not tolerate forgetfulness or slowness, or have much sympathy with emotional problems such as irritability or anxiety. Cognitive problems may mean that a person is unsafe to work with machinery, or though able to work, cannot do so quickly enough to be productive.

While the prospects of work for many are much reduced, it is important to bear in mind once again that few people in Britain receive any specialised rehabilitation focused on preparing them for work or providing them with new skills. Specialised work rehabilitation services for head-injured people are lacking, although the Department of Employment provides a general service to retrain all people with disabilities. An initial step is to apply for a course of employment assessment and rehabilitation. An application form can be obtained from a Job Centre which asks for an outline of past jobs and any medical problems. An assessment is then completed which may involve the injured person taking a number of psychological tests to see how quickly and accurately he or she can work, and what kind of job might be appropriate. The results of the assessment and the person's interests are considered, and a period of work experience and retraining may be arranged with a view to finding more permanent employment. When a compensation claim is being pursued a solicitor may arrange for a specialist vocational consultant to visit and assess the claimant's capacity for work and review what opportunities are available locally. He or she will write a report outlining the options that are available in the light of the person's physical and psychological condition, and this might involve recommending less demanding or part-time work, sheltered employment or advising that work is no longer possible. This report is primarily for use in legal proceedings, although it can nevertheless be used to guide thinking about what kind of work would be suitable.

Studying and education

Because the majority of people who have head injuries are either in their teens or early twenties many are still at school, college or university. Getting back to studying or training, however, may be difficult if there are cognitive and behavioural problems. When someone has had a severe head injury it may be readily apparent that he or she is no longer going to be able to cope with academic work or training. However, it may be much more difficult to predict how well someone with less serious injuries will cope. Subtle problems such as fluctuating concentration, slowness or a tendency to fatigue may render demanding academic work difficult, although these problems may not be otherwise particularly disabling. Unfortunately, schools and colleges often have little understanding of such problems and few have the experience or facilities to accommodate a head-injured student. It is therefore essential for the family to liaise closely with teachers as soon as possible and discuss any potential problems. Before the person returns to school an assessment may be completed either by a clinical psychologist or an educational psychologist (an educational psychologist is a psychologist specialised in assessing children's educational needs) and the views of other professionals such as a speech therapist, physiotherapist, occupational therapist and medical doctors may be sought. Usually a plan will be drawn up at a special meeting called a case conference which all the relevant people attend: the head-injured person and family, teachers, psychologist, and doctor. It may be agreed that a teacher should give home tuition and gradually reintroduce academic work to see how the head-injured person copes. Alternatively, it may be appropriate to return to school on a part-time basis, for mornings only say, and then gradually increase the amount of time at school. Some subjects may be dropped to ease the burden or extra tuition arranged after usual school hours. It may be that going back to an ordinary school is not successful, and that a move to a school for children with special needs is required. Dates will normally be agreed for everyone involved to review progress and check that the plan is working. Arrangements will also be set in place so that any problems that arise can be discussed at an early stage. Usually such a plan is not viewed as unchangeable but rather as a blueprint that can be altered and revised in the light of experience. Children of school age have a legal right to an education, and if they have a disability they are entitled to special provision, which can be enforced by law. If there are problems getting adequate provision these should in the first instance be taken up with the school or educational authority. An organisation to contact for advice is HIRE (Head Injury Re-Education) which promotes the educational needs of head-injured people and holds study days on head injury (address at the end of the book). Older students at college or university are not legally entitled to special educational provision although most academic institutions try to accommodate students' problems. A psychological assessment may be informative and highlight any cognitive problems before the young person tries to return. The psychologist may recommend taking time off from studying, a change of course or consideration of an alternative career path. Once again it is important to raise any problems with course tutors sooner rather than later, so that they can be discussed and arrangements made to help.

Living independently

There are a host of different aids for nearly all aspects of daily living which can make life easier for the disabled person. Before discharge from hospital an occupational therapist will usually assess how well each person copes with living independently and deals with domestic matters such as cooking, cleaning, paying bills and so on. This may involve a period of assessment in a hospital flat, where people who are soon to be discharged are asked to look after themselves overnight, cook and clean and generally run a household. If a person has difficulty coping, the occupational therapist will train him or her to maximise their capabilities and overcome the problem. The occupational therapist may also make a home assessment to see if there are any aids that might be needed and provide training in how to use them. The majority of aids are provided free of charge by local authorities. Throughout the country there are Disabled Living Centres where disabled people can go to view various aids and see them demonstrated. Professional advice is also available as well as information and training in their use. A list of Disabled Living Centres can be obtained from their central organisation, the Disabled Living Centre Council (address at the end of the book). Social services may also help with housing adaptations, and be able to advise on grants for any structural work. When someone's independence is compromised after head injury often this is not because of a physical handicap but because their judgement or memory is so poor that they would not be safe on their own. Distractibility or forgetfulness may place a person at risk because he or she might leave cooking unattended or fires on. In such circumstances even minor lapses of attention may have catastrophic consequences. Sometimes such problems can be overcome quite simply: using a microwave or an electric kettle with an automatic cut-out switch may, for instance, circumvent the risk of causing a fire due to forgetfulness while cooking. Of course, not all problems are overcome quite so easily. Impaired social judgement or an unwillingness or inability to appreciate one's limitations may mean that a person is susceptible to exploitation by unscrupulous people and it may not therefore be wise for them to live alone. Loss of insight may mean that a person is unwilling to take any special steps to ensure that they are safe. If a person is extravagant or disinhibited they may be unable to look after their finances properly or pay their bills. A clinical psychologist can assess these problems and, together with other colleagues such as an occupational therapist, make recommendations about the kind of living arrangements that would be suitable. It may be that it is no longer feasible to live alone, or a person's requirements are too great for their family and a move to sheltered accommodation is necessary. A social worker can advise on the options which are available locally and liaise with organisations such as the social services.

Cognitive assessment

Resuming independent living may be difficult for someone with cognitive problems. Some problems may be readily apparent, and it is sometimes quite clear simply from talking to a person that he or she has difficulties which preclude living alone or working. However, often these problems are not so clear-cut and indeed they may be quite subtle, yet in their own way no less disabling. A slight tendency to slowness or mild forgetfulness may not cause many difficulties at home, although it might prevent high-level intellectual study or work. To determine the exact nature of such problems and plan for the future it may be helpful to see a clinical psychologist to have what is known as a cognitive assessment. A cognitive assessment involves taking tests assessing concentration, memory, and problem-solving skills, as well as an evaluation of the ability to understand and produce speech, read, write, and copy. The psychologist will also be interested in determining how well a person is coping more generally and will ask questions about problems such as irritability and other emotional difficulties. Usually the psychologist will be interested in interviewing a relative to get as full a picture as possible. He or she will aim to build a picture of a person's strengths and weaknesses which they can discuss together and use to make plans for the future. The psychologist may pinpoint subtle cognitive difficulties and forewarn of any problems that might arise, as well as suggest practical strategies to avoid them. A course of treatment may also be recommended for other problems such as feelings of depression or problems with temper. Unfortunately the number of psychologists is limited and relatively few are specialised in completing such assessments, although GPs will be aware of a local hospital department to which a referral can be made.

Driving

Driving allows independence and freedom and can be an important boost to confidence and morale. However, head injury can mean that because of either psychological changes or physical problems driving is not allowed by law, either temporarily or permanently. Physical injuries such as double vision or a visual field defect may preclude driving; if a person suffers from epilepsy driving is forbidden and a licence will only be restored if the epilepsy is well controlled and there have been no fits for a year. Driving may not be allowed even if a person does not suffer from epilepsy but a doctor considers that there is a risk of it developing in the future. Just as important as any physical limitations are cognitive problems such as slowness, fatigue and limited concentration. Such factors may reduce a person's reaction time, and when travelling at speed when every second counts, it may be more difficult to avoid a collision. Emotional problems such as an explosive temper, irritability and lack of insight may also mean that a doctor considers it unsafe for a person to drive and his or her licence will be withdrawn. Before driving it is important to discuss whether it is safe to do so with a GP, and contact the Medical Advisory Branch of the DVLC whose address is at the end of this book. Some people are required to stop driving either indefinitely or temporarily, or asked to complete a special driving assessment at a driving centre.

The future: what is needed?

As every head-injured person and relative knows, adequate, properly organised rehabilitation services for brain trauma are lacking in the National Health Service. Medical treatment at the acute stage immediately after injury is excellent, but thereafter care tends to be piecemeal and disorganised. Therapy for psychological problems in particular is rare and few people receive a comprehensive package of care. This poor state of affairs persists despite the fact that the problems of the head-injured have now been recognised for many years and several reports by different bodies such as the Royal College of Physicians, the British Psychological Society, the Medical Disability Society and the Royal College of Psychiatrists have called for the establishment of a national strategy for the head-injured. Unfortunately these calls have gone largely unheeded, and such care as there is has increasingly been provided by the private sector. Unfortunately the cost of private treatment is prohibitive and invariably limited to those funded by insurance settlements. While such provision meets the needs of some, inevitably only a minority of those who could benefit are likely to receive help. What is required is the establishment of a comprehensive system of care within the National Health Service.

What kind of care do we need? As we have seen, some of the most important obstacles to re-establishing personal relationships, living independently and returning to work are in fact the psychological changes after injury, rather than physical impediments. Rehabilitation for these problems should start as soon as possible after head injury and involve a major and co-ordinated input, not just from medical staff but often more importantly from psychologists, social workers, nurses, occupational therapists, physiotherapists and speech therapists. All professional staff require training in the unique problems head-injured people experience, and, as many problems are not alleviated rapidly, a long-term commitment by all professionals is essential. A network of services is required so that the rehabilitation initiated in hospital continues afterwards to reintegrate brain-injured people back into the community and help them resume past interests and activities as well as get back to work. Finally, the needs of families and carers must be met, as they often bear the brunt of head injury and can experience more problems than the head-injured person. Carers need to be involved with, and part of, the rehabilitation team from the start and they require support, advice, information and respite.

Unfortunately such provision is as yet only an aspiration for both families and professionals alike, despite the fact that in the last decade there has been an enormous growth in the development of rehabilitation and treatment programmes for cognitive and behavioural problems, particularly in North America. The development of these therapies is at an early stage and many treatment methods are not yet of proven effectiveness. Nevertheless, a growing number of research studies suggest that such treatments can bring about significant and worthwhile improvement. A recent study in Denmark, for example, found that a group of people with head trauma and strokes who completed an intensive course of neuropsychological rehabilitation managed to re-establish relationships with their partners, resume many of their past leisure activities and required less practical assistance with their daily affairs. In addition, although many remained unemployed, significant numbers did manage to get back to work. Rehabilitation therefore holds considerable promise and the challenge now is to establish such provision in the future. The increasing recognition of head-injured people's needs by health planners and governments is an encouraging development, although much remains to be done before this is translated into a comprehensive system of care. Families and head-injured people have a central role to play in this process by energetically raising the profile of head injury among the public and media, pressing for the provision of services locally and lobbying nationally for change.

Appendix 1
Useful addresses

Who can help?

There are several organisations that can provide invaluable help and support for head-injured people and carers and in the following pages we will list some of the main bodies. This is not an exhaustive list, and there may be local organisations who can also assist. GPs' surgeries, local libraries, social services, the local church, and other head-injured people are all potential sources of information and support.

The only national body for head-injured people and their families is **Headway** (**National Head Injuries Association**). Headway consists of a central organisation based in Nottingham and numerous local groups around the country which organise regular talks and money-raising and recreational events. Headway aims to promote the interests of the head-injured at both a local and national level. It also organises a number of Headway Houses which are units run for brain-injured people. The local meetings are an invaluable way of getting in contact with other people in a similar position, making friends and sharing experiences. Headway sells several useful books and pamphlets on head injury and a regular magazine, *Headway News*, is sent to members. Contact the Nottingham office for a membership form and to obtain the address of a local group:

> National Head Injuries Association (Headway)
> 7 King Edward Court
> King Edward Street
> Nottingham NG1 1EW
> 0115 924 0800

The **Carers' Association** provides information and support to people who are caring at home and aims to promote their needs to various bodies and the government. Contact their head office to obtain the address of a local branch:

> Carers' National Association
> 20/25 Glasshouse Yard
> London EC1A 4JS
> 0171 490 8818

Crossroads is a national organisation which aims to provide practical support to carers by providing a home carer. Also contact your local social services office which may be able to arrange respite care:

Crossroads
Association of Crossroads Care Attendant Schemes Ltd
10 Regent Place
Rugby
Warwickshire CV21 2PN
01788 573653

SPOD (Association to aid the Sexual and Personal relationships of people with a Disability) provides advice and information to disabled people to help with sexual and relationship problems:

Association to aid the Sexual and Personal relationships
of people with a Disability (SPOD)
286 Camden Road
London N7 OBJ
0171 607 8851

If you have difficulty understanding your benefit entitlements your local hospital may have a Welfare Rights Officer who can advise you. You can also contact a local branch of the **Citizens' Advice Bureaux**. Their central address is:

National Association of Citizens' Advice Bureaux
Middleton House
115–123 Pentonville Road
London N1 9LZ
0171 833 2181

If you have continuing problems with your health or medication or you are a relative who is finding the stress of caring too much, consult your GP. He or she can then assess what course of action to take, such as changing your medicine, making a referral to a hospital consultant or arranging counselling. Your GP can also arrange a referral to other services such as those of a clinical psychologist, community psychiatric nurse, physiotherapist or speech therapist.

If you need information or advice on practical aids such as wheelchairs and adapted utensils the **Disabled Living Centres Council** can provide the address of a Disabled Living Centre in your locality where you can view equipment. Their address is:

Disabled Living Centres Council
286 Camden Road
London N7 OBJ
0171 700 1707

If you would like to resume driving, discuss with your GP whether you are ready and able to drive under the law. You should also notify the **DVLC** of your accident and condition at the following address:

Medical Advisory Branch
Floor D6
DVLC
Swansea SA99 1TU
01792 783438

A useful organisation which provides information and advice for newly disabled people regarding facilities, benefits and addresses of other relevant organisations is **RADAR** (**The Royal Association for Disability and Rehabilitation**):

RADAR
The Royal Association for Disability and Rehabilitation
Unit 12
City Forum
250 City Road
London EC1V 8AF
0171 250 3222

An organisation concerned with promoting the educational needs of head-injured people, disseminating information and holding study days on head injury is **HIRE** (**Head Injury Re-Education**). Their contact address is:

Portland College (HIRE)
Nottingham Road
Mansfield
Notts NG18 4TJ
01623 792141

For help with finding a suitable solicitor to conduct a compensation claim contact the **Law Society** or the **Association of Personal Injury Lawyers**:

The Law Society
50–52 Chancery Lane
London WC2A 1SX
0171 242 1222

Association of Personal Injury Lawyers (APIL)
10a Byard Lane
Nottingham NG1 2GJ
01159 580585

A useful group for people with epilepsy is the **British Epilepsy Association** which provides information and advice and has a network of self-help groups:

British Epilepsy Association
Anstey House
40 Hanover Square
Leeds LS3 1BE
01132 439393

The **British Psychological Society** publishes a directory which is a 'yellow pages' of chartered psychologists and the services they provide, including those who specialise in neuropsychology. Contact their main office:

The British Psychological Society
St Andrew's House
48 Princess Road East
Leicester LE1 7DR
0116 254 9568

For information on speech therapists and their services contact the **College of Speech Therapists**:

The College of Speech Therapists
7 Bath Place
Rivington Street
London EC2A 3DR
0171 613 3855

In the United States, contact:

National Head Injury Foundation
1776 Massachusetts Avenue North West
Suite 100
Washington DC 20036
USA
001 202 296 6443

National Head Injury Association
484 Main Street
325 Worcester

MA 01608
USA
001 508 795 0244

In Australia, contact:

Head Injury Council of Australia
P.O. Box 82
Mawson A.C.T. 2607
Australia
06 290 2253

Appendix 2
Suggestions for further reading

Headway publishes several useful pamphlets on aspects of head injury (such as memory problems, personality change, driving and legal issues) which are well worth purchasing. The following books are written for families and are also available through Headway:

Head Injury: the facts, Dorothy Gronwall, Philip Wrightson and Peter Waddell (Oxford University Press, Oxford, 1991)

Living with Head Injury: a guide for families, Richard C. Senelick and Cathy E. Ryan (Rehab Hospital Services Corporation, 1991)